To. Dr. Hugo Benalcazar
Neurosurgical Resident
Northwestern University
Medical School
Evanston Hospital

Here's hoping that you find
this book helpful.

Jeffrey Cozzens MD
Christmas 1996

Approaches in Neurosurgery

Approaches in Neurosurgery

Central and Peripheral Nervous System

I. Mohsenipour, W.-E. Goldhahn, J. Fischer, W. Platzer,
and A. Pomaroli

With 305 color illustrations by W.-E. Goldhahn

1994
Georg Thieme Verlag Stuttgart · New York
Thieme Medical Publishers, Inc. New York

Univ.-Dozent Dr. med. I. Mohsenipour
Universitätsklinik für Neurochirurgie
Anichstraße 35, A-6020 Innsbruck, Austria

Prof. Dr. med. habil. W.-E. Goldhahn
K.-Kollwitz-Str. 72, D-04109 Leipzig, Germany

Univ.-Dozent Prim. Dr. med. J. Fischer
Neurochirurgische Abteilung
Oberösterreichische Landesnervenklinik
Wagner-Jauregg
Wagner-Jauregg-Weg 15, A-4020 Linz, Austria

Univ.-Prof. Dr. med. W. Platzer
Institut für Anatomie der Universität
Müllerstrasse 59, A-6010 Innsbruck, Austria

Univ.-Dozent Dr. med. A. Pomaroli
Institut für Anatomie der Universität
Müllerstrasse 59, A-6010 Innsbruck, Austria

Library of Congress Cataloging-in-Publication Data

Approaches in neurosurgery : central and peripheral nervous
system / I. Mohsenipour ... [et al.] : with 305 color illustrations by
W.-E. Goldhahn.
p. cm.
Includes bibliographical references and index.
1. Nervous system-Surgery. 2. Anatomy, surgical and topographi-
cal. I. Mohsenipour, I.
[DNLM: 1. Nervous System-surgery. 2. Surgery, Operative-
methods. WL 368 A652 1994]
RD593.A68 1994
617.4'8-dc20
DNLM/DLC
for Library of Congress   94-32117 CIP

Edited by A.M. Wild, FRCS, 16 Blakes Way, Eaton Socon,
Huntingdon, Cambs. PE199 3PU, Great Britain

Manuscript translated by Gerhard S. Sharon, 4525 Henry Hudson
Parkway, Riverdale, NY 10471, USA

Important Note: Medicine is an ever-changing science under-
going continual development. Research and clinical experience
are continually expanding our knowledge, in particular our knowledge of proper treatment and drug therapy. Insofar as this book
mentions any dosage or application, readers may rest assured that
the authors, editors and publishers have made every effort to
ensure that such references are in accordance with the state of
knowledge at the time of production of the book.

Nevertheless this does not involve, imply, or express any guaran-
tee or responsibility on the part of the publishers in respect of any
dosage instructions and forms of application stated in the book.
Every user is requested to examine carefully the manufacturers'
leaflets accompanying each drug and to check, if necessary in consultation with a physician or specialist, whether the dosage sched-
ules mentioned therein or the contraindications stated by the
manufacturers differ from the statements made in the present
book. Such examination is particularly important with drugs that
are either rarely used or have been newly released on the market.
Every dosage schedule or every form of application used is entirely at the user's own risk and responsibility. The authors and
publishers request every user to report to the publishers any dis-
crepancies or inaccuracies noticed.

Cover drawing by Renate Stockinger, Stuttgart

© 1994 Georg Thieme Verlag, Rüdigerstrasse 14,
70469 Stuttgart, Germany
Thieme Medical Publishers, Inc., 381 Park Avenue
South, New York, NY 10016

Typesetting by
Hofacker DDV, Schorndorf, Germany

Printed in Germany by
Druckerei Grammlich, Pliezhausen, Germany

ISBN 3-13-100241-7 (GTV, Stuttgart)
ISBN 0-86577-541-9 (TMP, New York)

1 2 3 4 5 6

Preface

In the professional life of a surgeon, continued success depends to a large extent on a constant striving to acquire further training. This is increasingly true in this age of computers and microsurgical techniques. However, the new knowledge being acquired is useless as a rule unless it is based on a secure understanding of the anatomy. Compared with the anatomical training required in the study of clinical medicine, surgical anatomy needs to expand continually; it involves the surgeon's own steady and continued activity. In the absence of a grounding in anatomy that can be used in any way that may be required, neither optimal evaluation of a computed tomogram nor a structurally guided operative procedure using the surgical microscope, endoscopes, and microinstrumentarium, is possible.

The planning and execution of the approach have a critical role among the various phases of an operation. The smaller the approach, the greater the need for precise planning to avoid missing the target or causing „field injury."

For these reasons, the authors have joined in the effort to analyze the approaches commonly used for neurosurgical operations at their clinics and to describe these approaches in color illustrations with a concise narrative. They have deliberately confined themselves to their own personal knowledge and experience. Experienced surgeons will develop other approaches on their own initiative, but those who are still learning need to have a clear presentation of the standard operations. With an eye toward younger surgeons, too, we have chosen approaches with relatively large dimensions. As surgeons gain more experience, they will be able to reduce the size of the approaches themselves.

This book could not have been created without the personal and generous support of the project by Dr. med. h.c. Günther Hauff, Mr. Achim Menge, and their associates at Thieme. For this we wish to express our most heartfelt appreciation.

Innsbruck, Leipzig, and Linz   The authors

Table of Contents

Table of Contents

Table of Contents

The Organization of this Book and How to Use It

The text, captions, and illustrations are coordinated with each of the approaches discussed, so that the information provided may be either brief and concise or more detailed.

All the approaches are shown on the right side of the body; a quick conversion to the left-sided image can be obtained by turning over a copy made on a transparent sheet.

The illustrations represent the operative field as it is seen by the surgeon; not infrequently, therefore, broad side views are used. Each initial illustration shows the possible positioning of the patient, as well as one or more incisions that may be employed; the text then identifies the incision actually chosen. Special care has been taken to mark midlines.

The choice of colors is designed to enhance and clarify the information; they are not the natural colors, but are mutually comparable.

Proper names have been omitted both in the anatomical and neurosurgical terminology; the anatomical names used intentionally follow normal English-language usage.

References to the literature are given only for further reading, and are not intended to be complete or exhaustive. The authors remain well aware of other contributions made in the more distant past and in many related areas.

The very comprehensive subject index should serve to broaden and speed the reader's access to the available data.

1 Approaches to the Frontal Base

Unilateral Intradural Approach to the Frontal Base

Typical Indications for Surgery

— Cerebrospinal fluid fistulas secondary to frontobasal skull fractures
— Olfactory groove tumors, e.g., meningiomas
— Opening of the orbital roof
— Frontobasal angiomas

Principal Anatomical Structures

Auriculotemporal nerve, superficial temporal artery and vein, zygomatico-orbital artery, temporal fascia, temporoparietal muscle, frontal bone (squama), frontal tuber, coronal suture, frontal sinus, middle meningeal artery, frontal diploic vein, dura mater, falx of cerebrum, superior and middle frontal gyrus, superior sagittal sinus, bridging veins, frontal branches of anterior cerebral artery, frontal bone (pars orbitalis), crista galli, cribriform lamina, ethmoidal cells, sphenoid bone.

Positioning and Skin Incisions
(Fig. 1)

The patient is placed in supine position, and the head is turned to the contralateral side by 10–25 degrees, the greater degree of rotation being required for a unilateral incision.

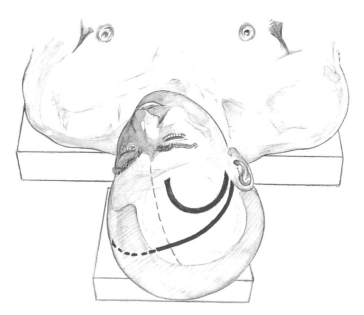

Fig. **1** Unilateral intradural approach to the frontal base. Positioning and incisions (arcuate incision and horseshoe incision)

Firm fixation of the head is required for the fine detail involved in the operative procedure. The head is not inclined, but instead slightly raised, to ensure adequate exposure of the frontal base.

A bilateral horseshoe incision is made, not only for cosmetic reasons, but also because the midline may be passed in the craniotomy.

With the usual hairline, and when there is no need to pass beyond the midline, the arcuate incision extends into the frontal hairline, notably on the right side.

Finally, it is also possible to opt for an incomplete horseshoe incision, which passes the midline but does not extend to the contralateral ear. The figures show exposure using the U-shaped incision.

Craniotomy
(Fig. 2)

After retraction of the galea aponeurotica and the periosteum, one or more burr holes are made in the squama of the frontal bone. Use of several burr holes is recommended if the approach is to extend to the superior sagittal sinus. Otherwise, the burr hole is placed in the dorsolateral angle; the bone flap is formed by passing the bone burr obliquely after retracting the dura from the bone with a Braatz probe. Despite the use of this probe, the dura may be injured, even with the use of the well-proven Gigli saw. Oblique passage of the burr or wire saw is designed to improve the stability of the reimplanted bone flap.

Opening the Dura
(Fig. 3)

The dura mater is opened in the direction of the longitudinal sinus. A clearance of several millimeters should be allowed between the bone margin and the dural incision, to facilitate the final closure of the dura. Full utilization of the craniotomy opening is made possible by tangential incisions at the corners. The actual dural flap may be left in place to serve as natural protection for the exposed frontal lobe pole. When it is reflected, special attention should be paid to the patency of the superior sagittal sinus. Elevation and retraction of the frontal lobe pole will subsequently expose the target area at the frontal base of the skull.

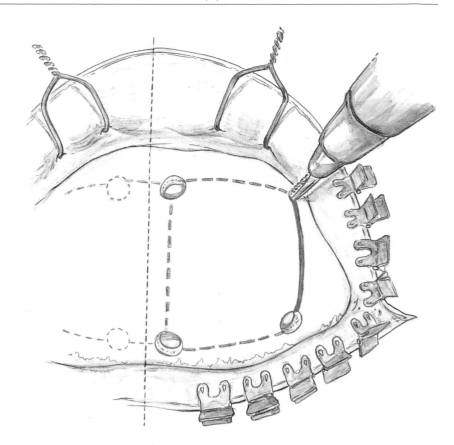

Fig. **2**   Horseshoe incision of the skin. Unilateral craniotomy with added burr holes alongside the superior sagittal sinus, and suggested possible expansion of the craniotomy to the contralateral side

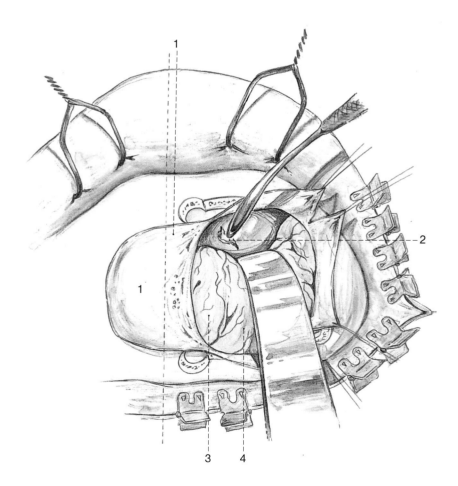

Fig. **3**   Development of the intradural frontal base and exposure of a frontobasal dural injury (cerebrospinal rhinorrhea)

1   Opened dura mater
2   Dural defect at bottom of the anterior cranial fossa
3   Superior frontal gyrus
4   Middle frontal gyrus

Within this frontal base, the exact position and extension of the ethmoidal cells play an important part in the planning of the operation (Fig. 4). In this regard, radiographs and computed tomography, with or without bone windows, are especially useful.

Dissection in the Area of the Superior Sagittal Sinus

(Fig. 5)

Technical problems may arise in the vicinity of the longitudinal sinus, either as a result of injury, or owing to lacunar evaginations of the sinus or bridging veins. When veins close to the sinus are exposed, a decision on whether to spare them should be taken with great care, so as to avoid the additional hindrance of cerebral edema developing in the course of the operation; the same considerations apply to postoperative complications. If a bridging vein can or must be divided, the bipolar coagulation is performed at a sufficient distance from the sinus (4–8 mm), and the division is made between two coagulation sites. If there has only been a slight injury to the vein where it enters the longitudinal sinus, application of hemostatic gauze (e.g., Tabotamp) generally proves more effective than bipolar coagulation directly at the sinus. The latter may lead to a larger sinus defect necessitating ligation.

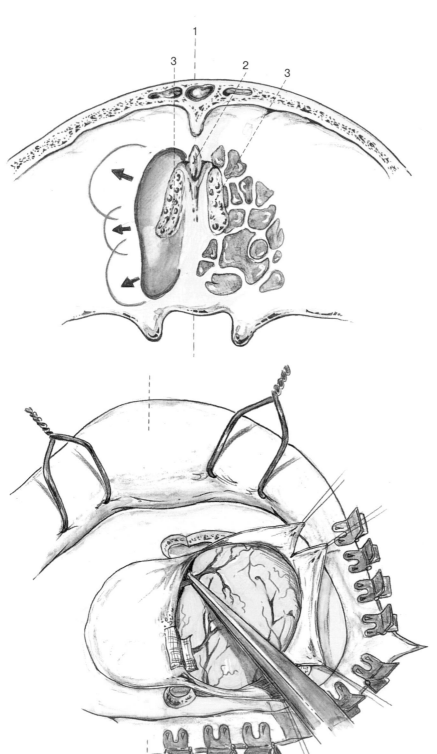

Fig. **4** Anatomical relations in the frontal base, diagrammatically on the left and on the basis of computed tomography on the right. The ethmoidal cells play a major role

1 Midline
2 Crista galli
3 Cribriform plate

Fig. **5** Securing veins near the sinus by bipolar coagulation or application of hemostatic fabrics, or both

Care of Injuries to the Superior Sagittal Sinus
(Fig. 6)

Since retention of venous drainage from the brain is as important as maintaining the arterial supply, ligation of a sinus should nevertheless always represent the last surgical resort. In the particular approach required for this indication, exposure of the bleeding site is usually readily feasible. With the bleeding contained using cottonoid sponges and suction, hemostasis is achieved so that a suitable section of muscle can be removed and two sutures may be passed in a U-shape through the falx and the dural flap. After this, the sponge is replaced by the muscle fragment, and the tension sutures may be tied over the muscle. During final closure of the dura, this reconstruction should be reexamined to make certain that the closure of the sinus lesion will not rebleed owing to diminution of dural tension.

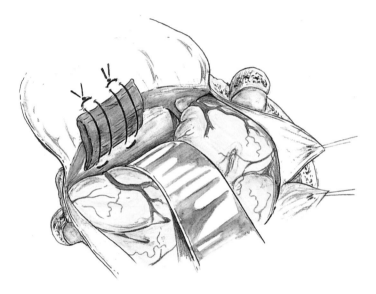

Fig. **6**   Repair of injury to the superior sagittal sinus by oversewing a muscle fragment

Dura, Bone, and Wound Closure

The dura is generally closed with interrupted sutures; a continuous suture may be used as well, but this would then have to be tied intermittently.

In the next step, the dural elevation sutures, which are best passed through indigenous bone channels, are tied, to minimize the risk of postoperative epidural hematomas. The same purpose is served, as is fixation of the bone flap, by U-sutures — also passed through the bone — at the center of the craniotomy, and these are tied over the bone flap. Together with the oblique bone incision, this provides for solid fixation at the craniotomy site. This fixation can be reinforced by means of tension sutures that are passed from adjacent periosteal regions over the bone flap.

Finally, the skin wound is closed with interrupted sutures after once more verifying subcutaneous hemostasis. If necessary, a suction drain can be placed, and the drain is brought out of the operative field via an adjacent stab incision.

Potential Errors and Dangers

— Overlooked loss of blood due to inadequate hemostasis in the cutaneous region
— Injury to the superior branches of the facial nerve when the skin incision has gone too far in the basal (temporal) direction
— Injury to the dura by craniotomy instruments
— Sinus injuries caused by craniotomy instruments
— Lesions to the brain and sinus due to unduly vigorous use of brain spatulas
— Tears in bridging veins
— Postoperative epidural hematoma due to inadequate or slack dural elevation sutures
— Soft-tissue hematoma due to inadequate hemostasis in the cutaneous region

Bilateral Extradural and Intradural Approach to the Frontal Base

Typical Indications for Surgery

- Olfactory groove meningiomas
- Special localizations of tumors in the chiasmatic region
- Hypothalamic tumors
- Frontobasal craniocerebral injuries
- Paranasal sinus tumors extending into the skull base
- Cosmetic corrections at the anterior skull base

Principal Anatomic Structures

Auriculotemporal nerve, superficial temporal vein and artery, zygomatico-orbital artery, temporal fascia, temporo-parietal muscle, supraorbital branch of the trigeminal nerve, supraorbital foramen or incisure, frontal bone (squama), superciliary arch, glabella, frontal tuber, coronal suture, frontal sinus, frontal diploic vein, middle meningeal artery, dura mater, falx of the cerebrum, superior and inferior sagittal sinus, bridging veins, frontal branches of the anterior cerebral artery, arteria pericallosa, frontal bone (pars orbitalis), crista galli, cribriform lamina, ethmoidal cells, sphenoid bone, olfactory bulb and tract, gyrus rectus.

Positioning and Skin Incisions
(Fig. 7)

The patient is placed in a supine position, with the head in a median position and slightly raised. Depending on the loca-

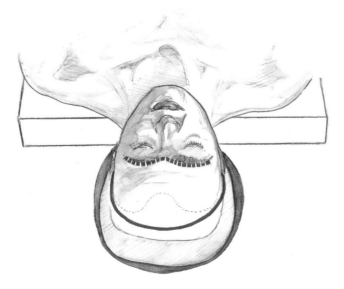

Fig. 7   Bilateral extradural and intradural approach to the frontal base. Positioning and incisions (border-of-eyebrow incision and horseshoe incision)

tion of the skin incision and the desired depth of the approach, the head may be slightly to markedly inclined. Fixation of the head is preferable in the majority of these operations, particularly if use of the surgical microscope is planned.

The neurosurgeon's preferred incision is U-shaped, from the beginning of one ear to the other. Rhinosurgeons not infrequently use the bilateral eyebrow incision. Since teamwork is advisable at all times, combinations of these incisions may be employed as well. It is important to note that the eyebrows are never shaved off in any operation.

Craniotomy
(Fig. 8)

A burr hole made dorsolaterally on the right side is theoretically sufficient. In actual practice, however, two burr holes near the longitudinal sinus are added, so that the dura in the sinus region can be dissected from the bone with maximal safety, thus avoiding a sinus injury. The dura in the area of the burr holes is dissected with the use of variously curved Braatz probes. This is done with particular care over the sinus region.

The actual bone flap can be cut with Gigli wire saws or with the craniotome, care being taken to make the cut oblique so that at the end of the operation the bone flap can be firmly anchored in the craniotomy opening. The bone flap is detached from the subjacent dura with blunt elevators, special caution again being taken in the sinus region. After removal of the bone flap, there is bleeding from small communicating veins to the sinus; cotton sponges impregnated with hot saline are applied here, followed by absorbable hemostatic gauze (e.g., Tabotamp).

Extradural Exposure of Frontal Base
(Fig. 9)

Once the sinus region has been secured, careful retraction of the dura-covered frontal lobe poles can begin. With the use of the slender Killian elevator, this can generally be accomplished without serious lesions or hemorrhages. The retraction of the brain has to be done with as much delicacy as in the intradural exposure, because the dura provides only limited protection from the edges of a spatula. The viewable area of frontal base depends on the extent of the exposure, and may therefore range from rather small to a considerable size, and it is by no means necessarily symmetrical.

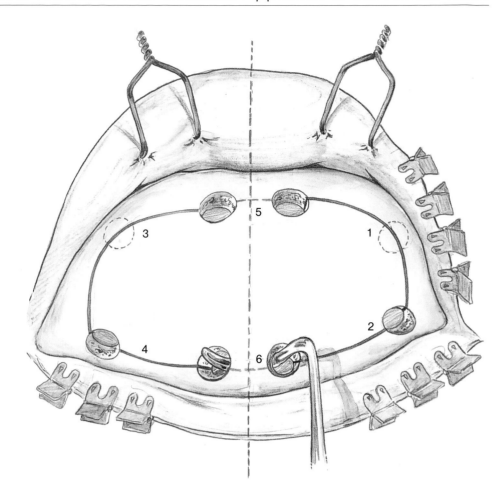

Fig. **8** Bilateral craniotomy en bloc, passing the superior sagittal sinus. The numbers indicate the order of the saw incisions required

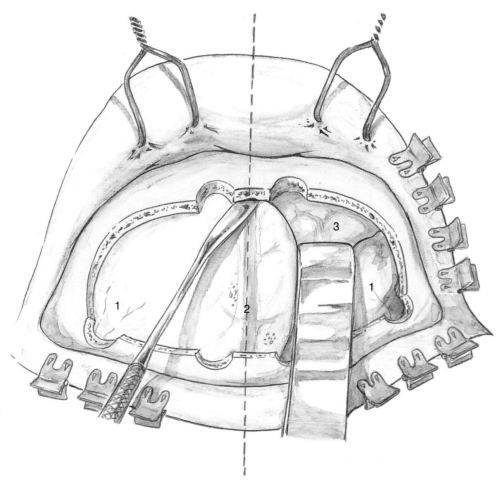

Fig. **9** Extradural development of the frontal base. The brain remains covered by dura

1 Dura mater with frontal branch of middle meningeal artery
2 Superior sagittal sinus
3 Orbital plate of the frontal bone, with protruding orbital roof

Intradural Exposure of Frontal Base
(Fig. 10)

Bilaterally developed pathological processes and structures extending deeply in the direction of the hypothalamus require an intradural procedure with transection of the sinus and falx. This is begun by a typical incision of the dura, somewhat removed from the border of the craniotomy and based with a posterior pedicle; the incision is made symmetrically on both sides. For full utilization of the craniotomy, relief incisions with elevation sutures are placed in the corners. At the superior sagittal sinus (Fig. 11), a moderate retraction of the brain is needed for visualization of the falx below the sinus. This makes it possible to pass two sutures, under vision, to the contralateral side under the sinus and to tie them over the sinus. Between these two ligatures, lying about 1.5 cm apart, the falx can be divided down to its inferior border (Fig. 12); spatulas ensure protection of the brain. As a rule, the inferior longitudinal sinus produces little or no bleeding, so that bipolar coagulation is sufficient. Complete transection of the falx provides the surgeon with an excellent overview of the frontal base.

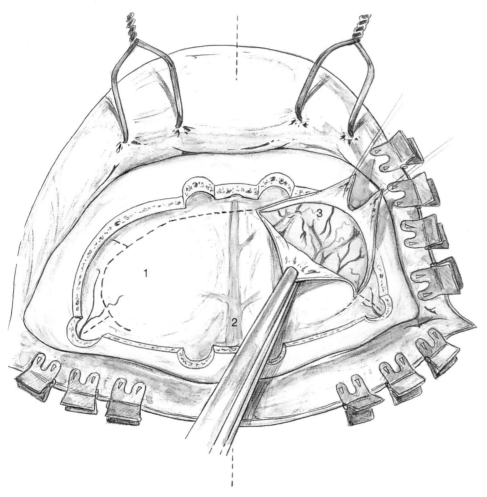

Fig. **10** Direction of the dural incision for bilateral intradural exposure of the frontal base

1 Dura mater
2 Superior sagittal sinus
3 Frontal pole

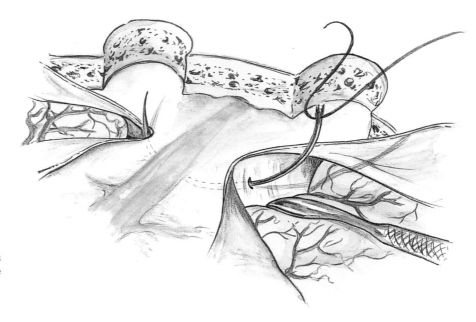

Fig. **11** Planned ligation of the superior sagittal sinus near its frontal end. Under vision, the sutures are passed through to the contralateral side in the falx below the sinus

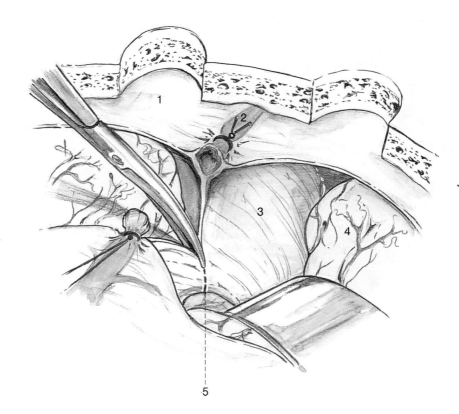

Fig. **12** The sinus ligatures are tied, the longitudinal sinus is divided, and the Cooper scissors cut through the adjoining segments of the frontal cerebral falx

1 Dura mater
2 Ligated and transected longitudinal sinus
3 Falx cerebri
4 Frontal pole
5 Inferior margin of the falx, with the inferior sagittal sinus

Intradural Development of the Frontal Base
(Fig. 13)

Retraction of the two frontal lobe poles is combined with a slight elevation; the spatulas are separated from the brain with the aid of cottonoid sponges, rubber, or (most naturally) with the dural flap. The self-retaining hooks generally used can only be applied with slight pressure, and should not be too narrow. Again, the scope of the frontal base exposure depends on the location and extent of the pathological process.

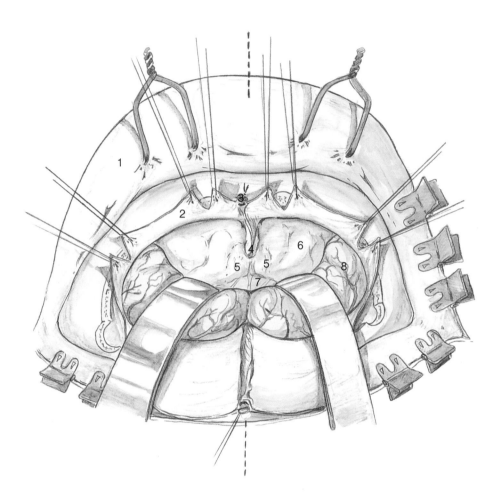

Fig. **13**   The dura-invested frontal base is bilaterally visualized after elevation and retraction of the frontal poles. The dural flap can be left on the brain for protection

1   Galea aponeurotica
2   Dura mater
3   Divided superior sagittal sinus
4   Crista galli
5   Cribriform lamina (covered by dura)
6   Orbital part of frontal bone
7   Prechiasmatic cistern
8   Frontal lobe of brain

Wound Closure
(Figs. **14, 15**)

Illustrated here is the creation of a galeal-periosteal flap using Dietz's method, which is most commonly used for extensive dural injuries secondary to frontobasal trauma. To this end, the anteriorly reflected skin flap is used to form an adequately sized galeal flap with a wide base (blue), which is stitched and glued onto the inside of the frontobasal dura. The previously reflected dura of the frontal lobe poles (red) is once again sewn to this layer with interrupted sutures. This is one of the safest means of closing extensive frontobasal cerebrospinal fluid fistulas and frontal sinuses.

In the next step, dural elevation sutures are placed and tied, preferably being passed through indigenous bone channels.

Via central bone channels and appropriate dural elevation sutures passed through these channels, the bone flap can be secured in its bed. The anchoring is reinforced by longitudinal placement of sutures in the galea and periosteum.

As a rule, bilateral suction drains, brought out via stab incisions in the vicinity, become necessary, as there may be rebleeding of the large wound surfaces even after careful hemostasis.

Potential Errors and Dangers

— Overlooked loss of blood due to inadequate hemostasis in the area of the skin flap
— Injury to branches of the facial nerve when a horseshoe incision extends too far basally
— Injury to the supraorbital branch of the trigeminal nerve from the marginal eyebrow incision (often unavoidable)
— Dural injury due to craniotomy instruments
— Sinus injury due to craniotomy instruments
— Inadequate hemostasis of the superior sagittal sinus and afferent bridging veins
— Brain lesion due to overly rigorous application of brain spatulas
— Bilateral rupture of the olfactory nerve (frequently a consequence of the preceding frontobasal trauma)
— Postoperative epidural hematoma due to inadequate or slack dural elevation sutures
— Soft-tissue hematomas due to inadequate hemostasis in the cutaneous region, absence of suction drains, and underestimation of the compression bandage

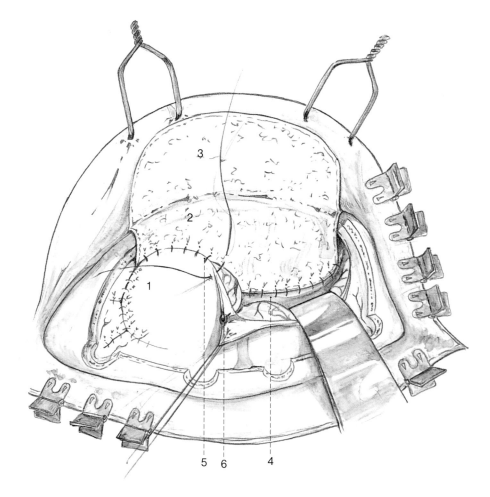

Fig. **14** Formation of infolded, pedicled galeal flap for sealing sizable frontobasal dural defects (Dietz procedure) and final suture of the frontal dura onto the inside of this flap

1 Frontal dura mater
2 Infolded galeal flap, with wide stalk toward the site of removal
3 Site of removal of the pedicled flap
4 Sutures between the infolded galeal flap and the basal dura mater
5 Dura-flap sutures over the frontal pole
6 Ligated superior sagittal sinus

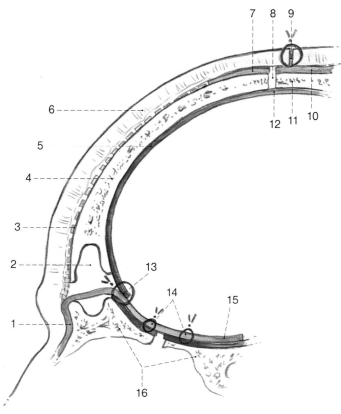

Fig. **15** Diagram of dural closure with the aid of an infolded galeal-periosteal flap (Dietz procedure)

1 Galea-periosteum at the nasion
2 Frontal sinus
3 Site of removal of galeal-periosteal flap
4 Frontal bone cover
5 Dura mater (red)
6 Frontal skin
7 Galea-periosteum at superior margin of bone cover
8 Craniotomy edge
9 Skin suture
10 Galea-periosteum
11 Parietal bone
12 Dura mater
13 Suture between the infolded galeal-periosteal flap and the inferior border of the dural flap
14 Sutures between the infolded galeal-periosteal flap and the basal dura mater
15 Infolded dural-periosteal flap (blue)
16 Frontal base

Paraorbital Transsphenoidal Approach to the Sella Turcica

Typical Indications for Surgery

— Intrasellar pituitary adenomas
— Intrasellar and locally suprasellar pituitary adenomas
— Craniopharyngiomas with sellar involvement
— Median frontal cerebrospinal fluid fistulas secondary to trauma and in cases of empty sella

Principal Anatomical Structures

Angular artery and vein, dorsal artery of nose, supratrochlear artery, supraorbital artery, supratrochlear nerve, supraorbital branch of the trigeminal nerve, orbicular muscle of the eye, occipitofrontal muscle (venter frontalis), corrugator supercilii muscle, orbital septum, adipose body of the orbit, trochlea, superior oblique muscle of the eyeball, frontal bone (pars nasalis and pars orbitalis), nasal bone, supraorbital incisure (foramen), anterior ethmoidal foramen, anterior and posterior ethmoidal cells, ethmoid bulla; superior, middle, and common meatus of the nose; perpendicular lamina of the ethmoid bone, vomer, superior nasal concha, sphenoidal sinus, sella turcica.

Positioning and Skin Incision
(Fig. **16**)

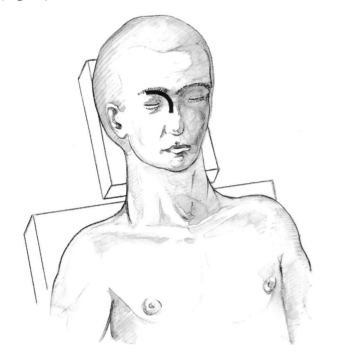

Fig. **16**   Paraorbital transsphenoidal approach to the sella turcica: positioning and incision

The patient is placed in a semisitting position, with the legs slightly elevated. The head remains in a median position, or is turned to the right by 5–10 degrees. Rigid immobilization of the head is not necessary.

The next step comprises rectangular alignment of the mobile radiography machine (C-arc), as well as appropriate radiographic monitoring of optimal sellar positioning. After this, changes in the height of the operating table should be avoided; otherwise, a simultaneous change in the height of the radiography equipment will be necessary.

The skin incision begins in the middle third of the (unshaved) right eyebrow, tracking it and then turning to the lateral surface of the nasal bone. The aim, therefore, is to carry out as cosmetically inconspicuous a procedure as possible, but whether this can be accomplished is not always predictable with absolute certainty; keloids do develop in some patients.

Hemostasis in the loose adipose tissue is effected using bipolar coagulation, and with meticulous precision so as to minimize postoperative swelling of the eye.

Dissection of the Nasal Region
(Fig. **17**)

Following retraction of the soft tissues without exposure of the trochlea, use may be made of a special spreader, which is serrated medially and features a suitable, somewhat resilient blade laterally. This spreader is used to keep the adjacent portions of the orbit out of the operative field. The orbital fat, too, usually remains beneath the spreader blade. If it should nevertheless protrude alongside the blade, stabilization of the tissue, hence its retraction, can be attempted by means of small bipolar coagulations. The bone region that is shaded red in Figure **17** is removed with a microburr, or with a fine chisel and a fine punch, so that the nose is opened from the lateral side.

Evacuation of Paranasal Sinuses
(Fig. **18**)

The mucosal parts and the bony and cartilaginous portions of the internal nose, the ethmoid, and the sphenoid bone can now be successively removed with the aid of straight or slightly angulated grasping forceps. The attendant hemorrhages usually cease after removal of the mucosa; if not, bipolar coagulation is indicated. Since the anatomical conditions are not generally consistent with exact adherence to the midline, some neurosurgeons are assisted by a rhino-surgeon, since rhinosurgeons very frequently use this approach for other indications, and observing the virtual midline is a routine matter for them. Once the anterior wall of the sella has been reached, the neurosurgeon performs the remainder of the operation by himself.

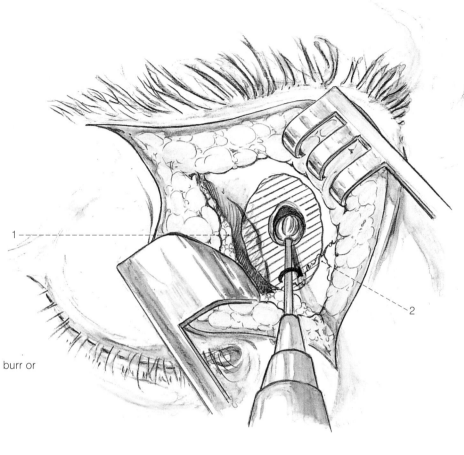

Fig. **17**   The lateral bony nose is opened with a burr or chisel (red-shaded area)

1   Orbital fat
2   Frontomaxillary and nasomaxillary suture

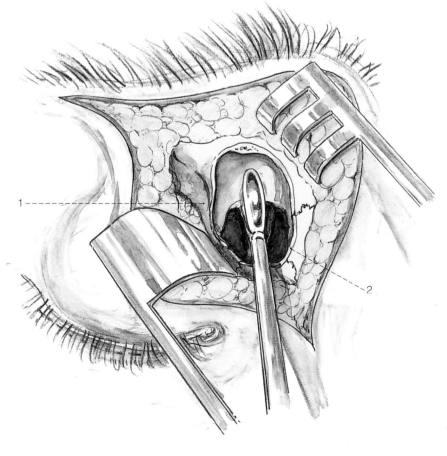

Fig. **18**   Removal of mucosa and osseous septa from the adjoining parts of the paranasal sinuses

Opening the Anterior Wall of the Sella
(Fig. **19**)

That the structure reached is indeed the anterior wall of the sella is verified by its typical appearance under the surgical microscope, and especially by radiography with the aid of the C-arc. A single method is not sufficient, since the radiographs are generally taken only from the lateral side.

As a rule, the bone of the anterior sellar wall is paper-thin, so that a fine chisel or the microburr quickly produces an opening for the micropunch. This punch removes the bone across a diameter of 8—12 mm; the lateral boundary can be visualized by a slight protrusion of bone over the carotid.

Opening the Intrasellar Capsule
(Fig. **20**)

The capsule tends to protrude slightly. After a cruciform or oval-shaped bipolar coagulation, it is incised with a very fine knife. The corners are turned outward. Hemorrhages from the capsular region, which not uncommonly communicate with the cavernous sinus, require bipolar coagulation with special forceps.

Exposure and enucleation of the tumor initiate the actual operation.

The adjacent structures to be watched are shown in Figure **21**.

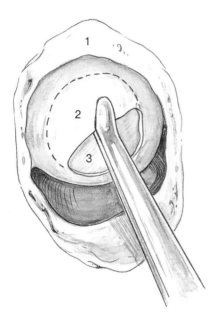

Fig. **19**   Ablation of the anterior wall of the sella after it has been opened with a microburr or a small chisel

1 Sphenoid bone
2 The anterior wall of the sella turcica to be opened, the sella having been widened by the tumor located behind it
3 Capsule of intrasellar tumor

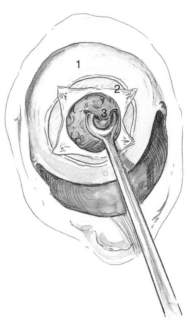

Fig. **20**   Cruciform incision and opening of tumor capsule. Removal of the tumor tissue can now begin

1 Sella turcica
2 Tumor capsule, opened and reflected
3 Tumor tissue

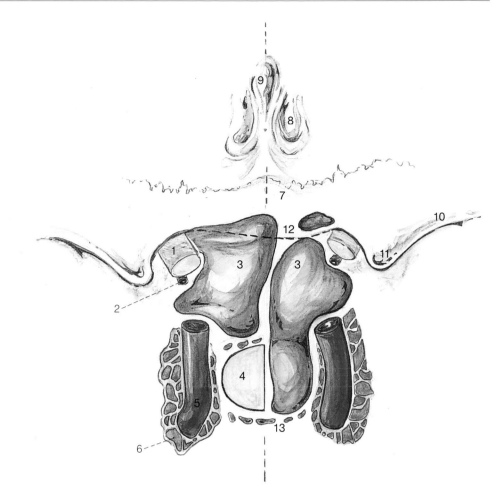

Fig. **21** Diagram of contiguous anatomical relations in the paraorbital transsphenoidal approach to the sella turcica

1 Optic nerve
2 Ophthalmic artery
3 Sphenoidal sinus
4 Left half of the pituitary gland
5 Internal carotid artery
6 Cavernous sinus
7 Sphenoidal plane with sphenofrontal suture
8 Cribriform plate
9 Crista galli
10 Small wing of the sphenoid bone
11 Anterior clinoid process
12 Sphenoidal jugum
13 Intercavernous sinuses

Closure of the Anterior Wall of the Sella
(Fig. 22)

The authors use divergent procedures. Some use flat pieces of cartilage to cover the opening. Others prefer packing particles of dura or plastic beneath the bone margins, as shown in the illustration. If a communication with the subarachnoid cavity can be ruled out with certainty, packing — internally and anteriorly—with pieces of cellulose gauze or cellulose sponge (such as Tabotamp) suffices. If cerebrospinal fluid has leaked, tissue fibrin sealant is also applied.

Wound Closure

On withdrawing from the wound, another search for sources of bleeding has to be made. This applies especially to the extraosseous soft tissues. When there has been complete hemostasis, closure of the skin wound with interrupted sutures is all that is required. Drainage is not necessary, because there is internal communication with the nose.

Potential Errors and Dangers

— Inadequate hemostasis in soft tissues
— Deviation from the midline
— Injury to the internal carotid artery when this has a far median location (identification of this situation is made

through preoperative angiography or computed tomography)
— Injury to the cavernous sinus (due to the numerous variations of this sinus).

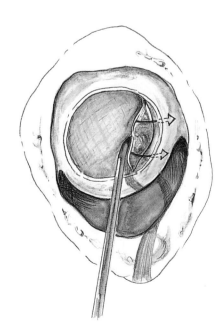

Fig. **22** Closure of the anterior wall of the sella with plastic material or thin bone

Transnasal Transsphenoidal Approach to the Sella Turcica

Typical Indications for Surgery

— Intrasellar pituitary adenomas
— Intrasellar and locally suprasellar pituitary adenomas
— Craniopharyngiomas with intrasellar involvement
— Selected clival tumors (e.g., chordomas)
— Tumors of the base of the skull with involvement of the sphenoidal sinus
— Injuries or hemorrhages in the sellar region
— Median frontobasal cerebrospinal fluid fistulas secondary to trauma, and in cases of empty sella

Principal Anatomical Structures

Anterior nasal spine, greater alar cartilage, cartilage of nasal septum, nasal muscles, perpendicular lamina of ethmoid bone, sphenoidal sinus and variations, sella turcica and variations, sellar diaphragm, clivus, carotid canal, cavernous sinus.

Positioning and Skin Incision
(Fig. 23)

The patient is placed in a semisitting position, and the head is extended by about 20 degrees. Rigid fixation of the head could be a hindrance, since it would hamper intraoperative adjustments of the position. Next, the mobile radiography unit (C-arc) is set up for lateral fluoroscopy. In addition to anesthesia, infiltration of the oral mucosa below the gingivolabial fold and mucosal infiltration of the cartilaginous nasal septum, e.g., with ornithine/vasopressin (Por 8; diluted 1:10), to minimize bleeding and facilitate dissection, are recommended.

Skin incisions per se are omitted, since incisions, both in the nose (Fig. **24a**) and in the mouth (Fig. **24b**), are made in the mucosa, which is bound to enhance the cosmetic outcome.

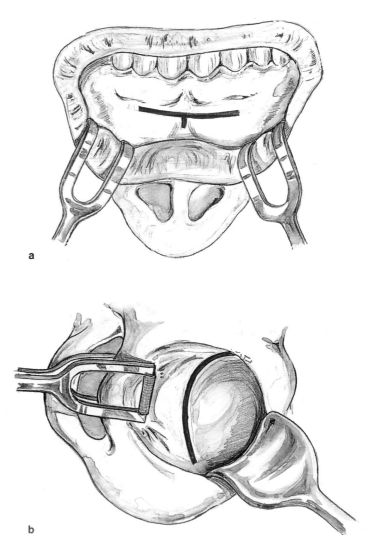

a

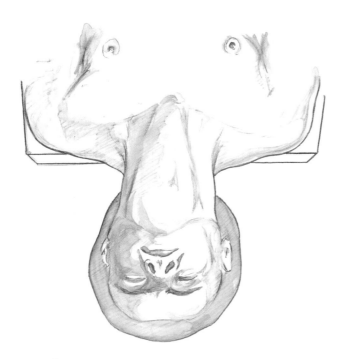

b

Fig. **23** Transnasal transsphenoidal approach to the sella turcica: positioning, with head dependent

Fig. **24** Incisions, **a** in the mouth, **b** in the nose

Dissection of Soft Tissues
(Fig. 25)

The mucous membrane and the periosteum have been incised over a length of 3–4 cm below the gingivolabial fold, exposing the piriform aperture through retraction of the periosteum. If need be, the Hajek punch may be used for inferior enlargement medially and laterally. This is followed by tunneling and dissection of the mucosa of the nasal floor and subsequent exposure of the superior margin of the cartilaginous septum and cautious tunneling of the perichondrium on one side of the nasal septum; laceration of the mucosa is to be avoided (Fig. 26). Sharp dissection at the perichondrial-periosteal interface occasionally becomes necessary in order to join the two tunneled pouches.

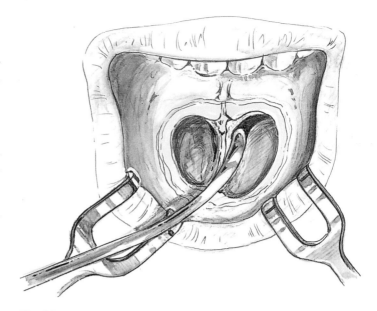

Fig. **25** Retraction of the nasal mucosa in the intraoral approach

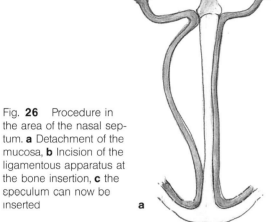
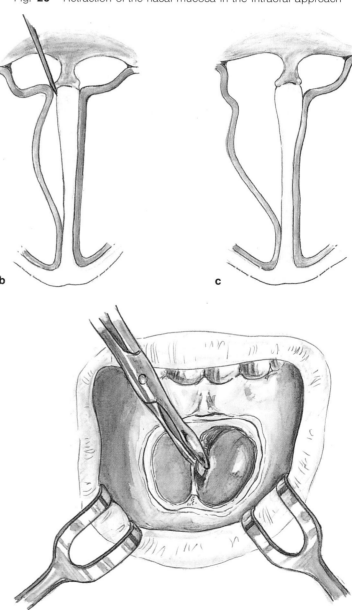

Fig. **26** Procedure in the area of the nasal septum. **a** Detachment of the mucosa, **b** Incision of the ligamentous apparatus at the bone insertion, **c** the speculum can now be inserted

Following sharp separation of the cartilaginous septum from the nasal spine, it is dislodged from the bony septum and divided at its boundary. The septal mucosa is carefully retracted to the opposite side, so that portions of the bony septum can be removed down to the wedge-shaped attachment at the floor of the sphenoid sinus (Fig. 27).

Fig. **27** Resection of small bony portions of the anterior nasal spine

Dissection of the Sphenoid Sinus
(Fig. 28)

A thin sphenoid sinus floor can easily be opened with rongeurs and rongeur forceps; if not, chisels and microburrs are used. Bleeding from the bone may necessitate impaction of wax, and hemorrhages from the mucosa require bipolar coagulation. After this, optimal use is made of the speculum, possibly following ablation of parts of the spina oris. At this point, the surgical microscope should be pivoted into position.

In the next step, the sphenoid sinus mucosa and septa that may be present in the sphenoid sinus can be removed. A hydrogen peroxide solution is still effective in stopping oozing hemorrhages. Identification of the median plane may prove difficult, so that turning of the C-arc becomes necessary. The paranasal sinuses show a pronounced asymmetry. Nor does the imaginary median line between the spina oris and the attachment of the osseous nasal septum at the nasal floor offer any absolute certainty. Protrusion of the sella turcica – which is quite substantial in a great many patients – due to pressure of the tumor is a more reliable indicator. This added means of orientation is not available if there is no enlargement of the sella.

Dissection in the Sellar Region
(Fig. 29)

In the majority of patients, the floor of the sella is very thin, and it can therefore be indented and ablated with a fine Hajek punch. A somewhat thicker sellar floor requires the use of fine chisels or microburrs prior to application of the punch. The exact positioning of the opening instruments is monitored using the laterally placed C-arc, as is the position of inserted instruments. When widening the gap in the floor of the sella, attention should especially be paid to the course of the internal carotid artery in its channel. Only in a few cases does a distinct furrow appear at the junction with the median, hence resectable, portion of bone. The distance between the two carotids should be determined during the preoperative examination; it may be very small. Portions of the cavernous sinus may be opened up in the vicinity of the bony resection area. The bleeding is initially controlled with hemostatic agents. Occasionally, the use of a specially developed bipolar coagulator that pushes the opened vessel against the border of the bony aperture becomes necessary. The normal bipolar forceps does not usually help, tending instead to enlarge the bleeding lesions.

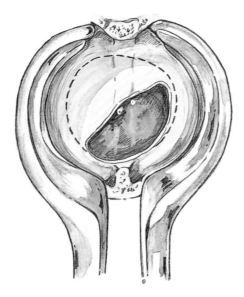

Fig. **28** The speculum has been inserted, the sphenoid septum ablated, and the anterior wall of the sphenoidal sinus partly resected

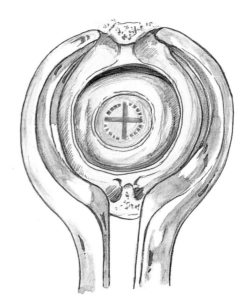

Fig. **29** The anterior wall of the sella turcica has been cut with the craniotome, and the cruciform or circular site of incision of the tumor capsule has been drawn in

The tumor capsule can be incised in a cruciform or annular fashion, the latter method being chosen if excision of capsule portions for histologic study is intended.

For the transnasal approach, only the first operative step needs to be altered, as shown in Fig. **24b**. Subsequent dissection follows the description given for the transoral procedure.

Wound Closure

Closure of the craniotomy opening in the floor of the sella is required mainly when escape of cerebrospinal fluid has been detected. For this purpose, a construct of lyophilized dura, fascia lata or similar material is inserted below the bony edges, and fixed with fibrin adhesives. Matching pieces are introduced into the sphenoid sinus with fibrin foam. The speculum can be removed, and the displaced osseous nasal septum reduced. The sublabial or intranasal incision site is closed with fine absorbable suture material, as are any lesions of the nasal mucosa. The nasal cavities are packed for two to three days with Vaseline strips.

Potential Errors and Dangers

— Missing the midline
— Injury to the carotid arteries in their bone channels
— Injury to the cavernous sinus
— Major injury to the nasal mucosa
— Nasal deformity due to excessive ablation of bony septum
— Postoperative bleeding and infection
— Persistent postoperative cerebrospinal fistula

2 Approaches for Operations in the Orbital Region

Subfrontal Intracranial Approach to the Orbit

Typical Indications for Surgery

- Tumors of the optic nerve, notably optic gliomas
- Tumors in the posterior portion of the orbit, notably meningiomas
- Decompression of optic nerve associated with treatment of a frontobasal injury

Principal Anatomical Structures

Auriculotemporal nerve, superficial temporal vein and artery, zygomatico-orbital artery, temporal fascia, temporo-parietal muscle, frontal bone (squama), frontal tuber, coronal suture, frontal sinus, middle meningeal artery, frontal diploic vein, dura mater, frontal bone (pars orbitalis), sphenoid bone (lesser wing and greater wing), ethmoid bone (cribriform lamina), crista galli, cecal foramen, optic canal, common tendinous ring (Zinn), optic nerve, frontal branch of trigeminal nerve, trochlear nerve, supratrochlear nerve, oculomotor nerve, nasociliary nerve, abducens nerve, lacrimal nerve, internal carotid artery, ophthalmic artery, anterior and posterior ethmoidal arteries, lacrimal artery, supratrochlear artery, supraorbital artery, rectus superior bulbi muscle, superior oblique muscle, superior ophthalmic vein, inferior and posterior ciliary veins, central artery and vein of retina, frontal lobe.

Positioning and Skin Incisions
(Fig. 30)

The patient is in a supine position, with the head slightly raised and turned to the right by 10–20 degrees. The 20-degree turn is used for a unilateral incision, and the smaller turn for a U-shaped (horeseshoe) incision. Firm fixation of the head is recommended.

The unilateral skin incision is made within the hairline; it is arcuate, and extends from 3 cm to the side of the midline to the superior anterior border of the ear. When there is a very high hairline, and for treatment in connection with a fronto-basal fracture, a U-shaped incision from the beginning of one ear to the other is preferred, but this incision need not always extend to the opposite ear. The figures show exposure using the unilateral skin incision.

Craniotomy
(Fig. 31)

With the use of a craniotome, a single dorsolaterally placed burr hole is sufficient. For the Gigli saw, several holes are required. In all cases, the dura, insofar as it is accessible, is retracted from the bone, starting at the burr hole. The incision by saw or craniotome should be made obliquely, so as to anchor the bone flap on reinsertion.

Dissection at the Base of the Skull
(Fig. 32)

The extradural procedure requires careful detachment of the frontal dura from the basal bone, using blunt, slender elevators. After this, the dura-covered frontal lobe pole may be raised with one or two spatulas and displaced posteriorly, so that the frontal base is brought into view. As a rule, its surface will display the more or less fissured texture of the orbital roof, from which the putative optic canal can be traced caudally. If the space is wide enough, the common tendinous ring (Zinn's ring) can be exposed and dissected into the optic canal with a slender punch. Otherwise, this canal is opened with a well-cooled microburr and fine punches at the posterior border of the orbital roof. In decompression associated with treatment of a frontobasal fracture, the resultant bone defect is narrower than in tumor trephination, which may well necessitate working dimensions of 20 to 30 mm.

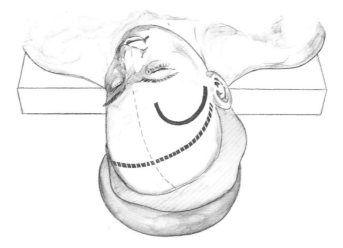

Fig. **30** Subfrontal intracranial approach to the orbit. Positioning and skin incisions (arcuate and horseshoe incisions)

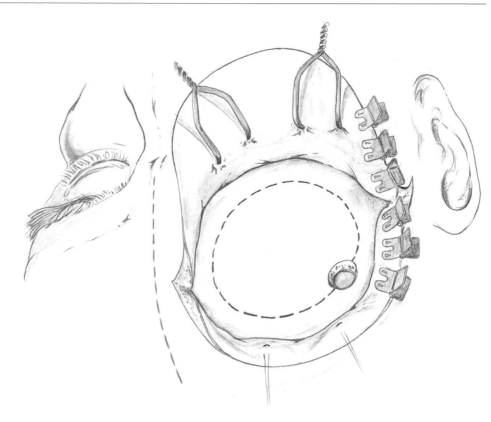

Fig. **31** Right-sided frontal craniotomy
following an arcuate incision. One burr hole
may be used, from which to cut the cranium.
Otherwise, several burr holes are connected
by incision with the Gigli wire saw

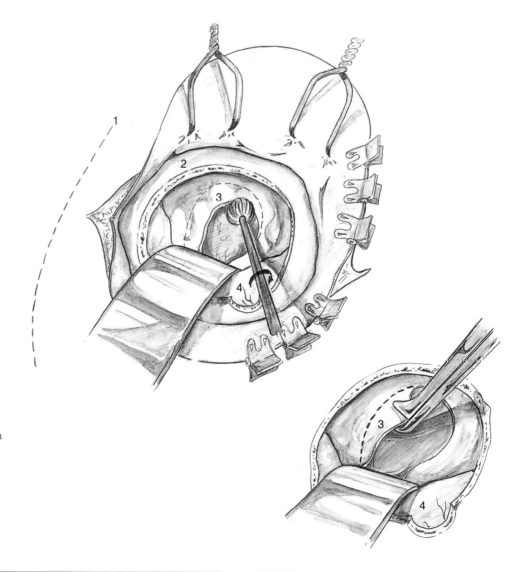

Fig. **32** Opening of the orbital roof after a
right-frontal osteoplastic craniotomy and
retraction of the dura-invested frontal lobe
pole. Use may be made either of a water-
cooled microburr or of fine punches

1 Midline
2 Frontal bone (squama)
3 Frontal bone (orbital part)
4 Frontal pole (covered with dura)

It is important to pay careful attention to the oblique course of the optic canal between the posterior wall of the eye and the optic chiasm (Fig. 33). Figure 33 also shows the course of the adjacent eye muscles.

If an intradural procedure is used primarily or secondarily, the arcuate, centrally based dural incision with tangential cuts is initially added to the steps described. Following elevation and reduction of the frontal pole, the basal dura is incised over the putative optic canal and retracted laterally. The ensuing procedure conforms to the extradural dissection described above.

Closure of Opening in Base of Skull
(Fig. 34)

Even though some type of orbital roof reconstruction is not necessary in all cases, and not with a narrow extradural dissection, one should be prepared to perform such a reconstruction. Many materials have been suggested and used for this purpose, ranging from tantalum plates to costal cartilage and soft structures. The latter, in the form of lyophilized dura, fascia, or plastics, usually prove adequate. The suitably trimmed material is inserted below the bone margins, or anchored to the bone with fibrin glue.

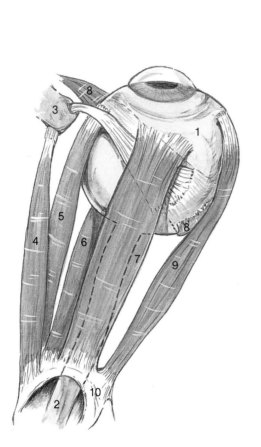

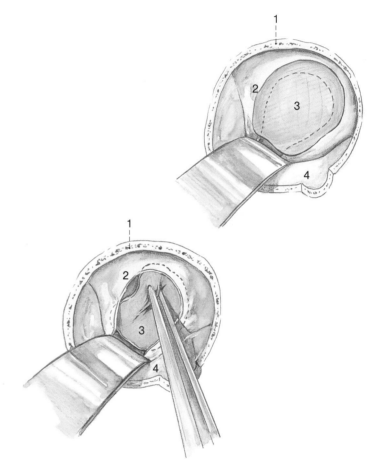

Fig. **33**   The eye, the optic nerve, and the ocular muscle, viewed from above

1   Eyeball
2   Optic nerve
3   Trochlea with tendon sheath of superior oblique muscle
4   Superior oblique muscle
5   Rectus medialis muscle
6   Rectus inferior muscle
7   Rectus superior muscle
8   Inferior oblique muscle
9   Rectus lateralis muscle
10 Common tendinous ring (Zinn)

Fig. **34**   Closure of the resected orbital roof. **a** Gluing-on of reconstruction material (Lyodura, plastics, etc.) **b** Reconstruction material is packed under the border of the orbital roof

1   Frontal bone (squama)
2   Frontal bone (orbital part)
3   Reconstruction material (green)
4   Retracted dura-invested frontal lobe pole

Wound Closure

In an intradural procedure, this operative step begins with the placement of interrupted sutures in the dura. Otherwise, the dura-covered frontal lobe pole merely needs to be replaced in its original position. Subsequently, dural elevation sutures – preferably passed through the indigenous bone channels – are placed for the purpose of preventing postoperative hematoma. The same purpose, as well as fixation of the bone flap, is served by central dural elevation sutures, which are likewise passed through directly overlying bone channels in the bone flap. If necessary, this flap may be anchored even more firmly by means of longitudinally placed tension sutures in the galeal periosteum.

Potential Errors and Dangers

— Overlooked loss of blood due to deficient hemostasis in the cutaneous region
— Injury to superior branches of the facial nerve due to excessive temporobasal extension of the skin incision
— Dural injury due to craniotomy instruments
— Brain lesions due to unduly vigorous application of the brain spatula
— Injuries to the eye muscles and nerves
— Postoperative epidural hematoma due to inadequate or slack dural elevation sutures
— Soft-tissue hematoma (subaponeurotic, to the upper eyelid) due to inadequate hemostasis in the cutaneous region.

Anterior Extracranial Superior Approach to the Orbit

Typical Indications for Surgery

— Intraorbital tumors at the superior and internal wall
— Mucoceles penetrating the orbit
— Circumscribed frontobasal lesions

Principal Anatomical Structures

Angular artery and vein, dorsal artery of the nose, supratrochlear artery, supraorbital artery, zygomatico-orbital artery, supratrochlear nerve, supraorbital branch of the trigeminal nerve, lacrimal nerve (superior palpebral branch), orbicular muscle of the eye (pars orbitalis), corrugator supercilii muscle, occipitofrontal muscle (venter frontalis), periorbita, frontal bone (pars nasalis and pars orbitalis), supraorbital incisure (foramen), sphenoid bone (greater and lesser wings); rectus superior, medialis and lateralis muscle; eyeball, lacrimal gland, superior ophthalmic vein.

Positioning and Skin Incision
(Fig. 35)

The patient is placed in a semisitting position, and the head is turned slightly toward the surgeon. The foot of the operating table is slightly raised. Firm fixation of the head is dictated by the need for extremely delicate maneuvers, and the position therefore depends on the precise location and the extent of the pathologic process.

The skin incision is made in, or a few millimeters below, the (unshaved) eyebrow. The choice of the exact location of the skin incision is determined by the local cosmetic requirements.

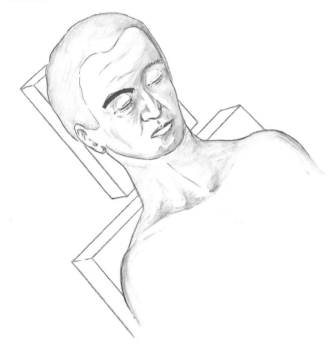

Fig. **35** Anterior extracranial superior approach to the orbit: positioning and incision

Dissection of the Superior Orbit

(Fig. 36)

After careful bipolar hemostasis within the fatty tissue, it is possible to expose the pars orbitalis of the orbicular eye muscle and the nerves and vessels coursing at the orbital border. The muscle fibers can be dissociated without great difficulty, the nerves and vessels remaining above the separating elevator. The layer being sought and maintained lies between the bone of the orbit and the periorbita.

A topside view of the anatomical relations, that is, in the specified area to be dissected, is presented in Figure 37.

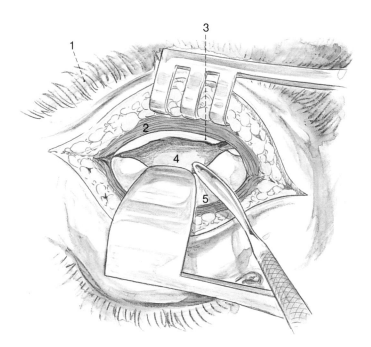

Fig. **36**   Retraction of the periorbita-covered orbital contents

1 Eyebrow
2 Orbicular muscle of the eye
3 Superior margin of the orbit, with the supraorbicular artery and nerve
4 Orbital roof from below
5 Periorbita

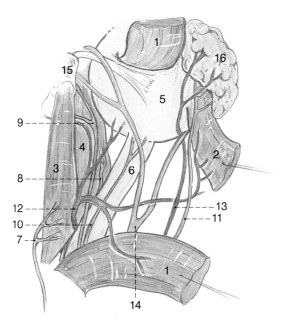

Fig. **37**   Anatomical representation of the orbital contents, viewed from above. The orbital roof, periorbita, and the levator muscle of the upper eyelid have been removed; the rectus bulbi superior muscle has been divided in the middle and reflected toward its ends

1 Rectus bulbi superior muscle
2 Rectus bulbi lateralis muscle
3 Superior oblique muscle of the eye
4 Rectus medialis bulbi muscle
5 Eye
6 Optic nerve
7 Trochlear nerve
8 Inferior branch of the oculomotor nerve
9 Nasociliary nerve and infratrochlear nerve
10 Long ciliary nerves
11 Lacrimal nerve
12 Ophthalmic artery
13 Lacrimal artery
14 Superior ophthalmic vein
15 Trochlea
16 Lacrimal gland

Dissection in the Superior Intraorbital Region
(Fig. 38)

By gradually retracting the sutures between the orbital bone and the periorbita, the surgeon reaches the middle and posterior portions of the orbital cavity. In Figures **33** and **37**, the highly vulnerable structures of the eye muscles and eye muscle nerves have been exposed. If the tumor is localized entirely outside the periorbita, this dissection can generally be accomplished without added damage. In the presence of infiltrative processes, on the other hand, such injuries – insofar as they are not caused by the underlying process itself – are often unavoidable. A special spreader, with blunt teeth at one end and a slightly resilient spatula blade at the other, is suitable for elastic retraction of the orbital contents.

Wound Closure

On leaving the depth of the operative site, another meticulous search is made for small sources of bleeding. Such sources are closed by bipolar coagulation, under good vision, so that damage to accompanying nerves can be avoided. Sutures are hardly needed except for approximation of the orbicular eye muscle. Use of a suction drain would be the exception.

In keeping with the cosmetic conditions, the skin is closed with fine interrupted sutures.

Potential Errors and Dangers

- It is a general rule not to shave eyebrows
- The skin incision should be optimally adapted to the cosmetic conditions
- Even the smallest hemorrhages should be controlled to avoid a substantial spread of hematomas across the loose tissue of the orbit and surrounding areas
- Dissection and coagulation require optimal vision and illumination, e.g., using the surgical microscope

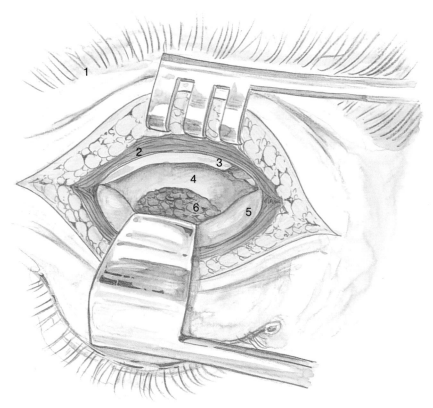

Fig. **38** Clarification of tumor in the area of posterior superior orbit

1 Eyebrow
2 Orbicular muscle of the eye
3 Superior border of the orbit, with the supraorbital artery and nerve
4 Orbital roof from below
5 Periorbita
6 Tumor

Anterior Extracranial Median Approach to the Orbit

Typical Indications for Surgery
— Tumors of the median orbital wall
— Mucoceles penetrating the median orbit

Principal Anatomical Structures

Angular artery and vein, dorsal artery of the nose, supra-trochlear artery, supraorbital artery, infratrochlear nerve, supratrochlear nerve, supraorbital branch of the trigeminal nerve, orbicular muscle of the eye, occipitofrontal muscle (venter frontalis), corrugator supercilii muscle, orbital septum, adipose body of the orbit, trochlea, superior oblique muscle, frontal bone (pars nasalis and pars orbitalis), nasal bone, supraorbital incisure (foramen), anterior ethmoidal foramen, anterior and posterior ethmoidal cells, ethmoid bulla; superior, middle and common meatus of the nose; perpendicular lamina of the ethmoid bone, sphenoid sinus.

Positioning and Skin Incision
(Fig. 39)

The patient is placed in a semisitting position, with the head turned slightly toward the surgeon and slightly raised. The foot of the operating table is slightly raised. Firm fixation is dictated by the location of the pathologic process and the anticipated delicacy of the dissection; therefore, it is frequently required.

The arcuate skin incision runs in or a few millimeters below the (unshaved) eyebrow, and extends as far as the lateral root of the nose, depending on the required size of the approach. The bony margin of the orbit is the guiding structure. The objective is to achieve as cosmetically inconspicuous a scar as possible; despite all efforts, however, this can by no means be assured – many patients develop keloids.

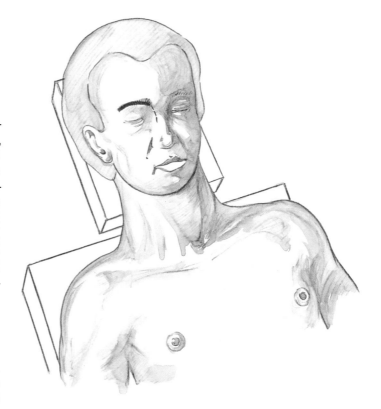

Fig. **39** Anterior extracranial median approach to the orbit: positioning and incision. *Dashed line:* possible extension

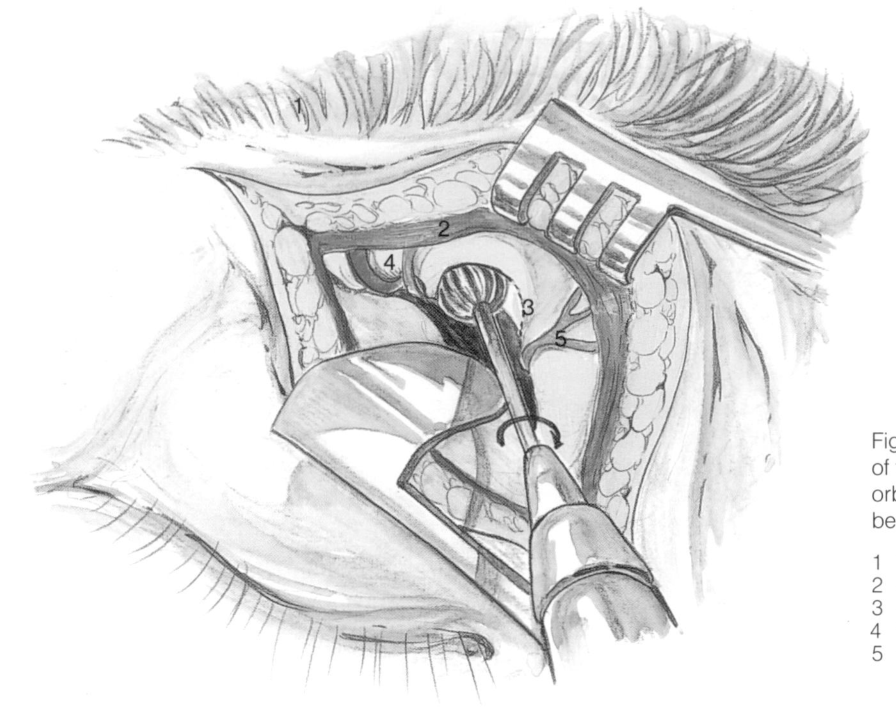

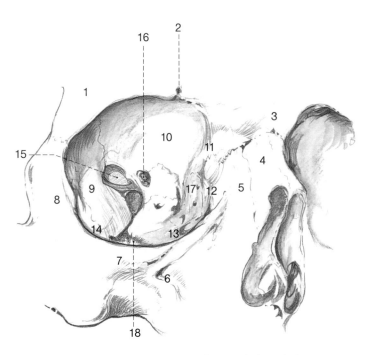

Fig. **40** The periorbita has been retracted. Visualization of the orbit interior is optimized by removal of small orbital border regions, many small nerves and vessels being retractable

1 Eyebrow
2 Orbicular muscle of the eye
3 Orbital border
4 Supraorbital artery and nerve (lateral branch)
5 Supraorbital nerve (medial branch)

Opening the Orbit with Minor Bone Resection
(Fig. **40**)

Careful bipolar hemostasis in the divided adipose tissue will give access to the pars orbitalis of the orbicular muscle of the eye, allowing it to be dissociated in the direction of the fibers. The overlying vessels and nerves are retracted, and are divided only if absolutely necessary. Using a microburr or fine chisel and fine punch, a crescent-shaped section of bone at the orbital margin, freed of periosteum, is removed in the direction of the floor of the ipsilateral frontal sinus, so that a straight view into the median orbit is provided.

After this, the space between the bones of the orbit and the periorbita is identified; in the presence of infiltrative processes the periorbita has to be opened.

Information about the osseous conditions in this orbital area is given in Figure **41**, and the adjacent lacrimal apparatus is presented in Figure **42**.

Fig. **41** Right bony orbit in a semioblique right frontal view

1 Frontal bone (zygomatic process)
2 Supraorbital incisure (foramen)
3 Glabella
4 Right nasal bone
5 Frontal process of the maxilla
6 Infraorbital foramen
7 Infraorbital margin
8 Zygomatic bone (frontal process)
9 Sphenoid bone (orbital surface, great wing)
10 Frontal bone (orbital surface of the orbital part)
11 Ethmoid bone (orbital lamina)
12 Lacrimal bone
13 Maxilla (orbital surface)
14 Zygomatic bone (orbital surface)
15 Superior orbital fissure
16 Optic canal
17 Ethmoidal foramina
18 Inferior orbital fissure

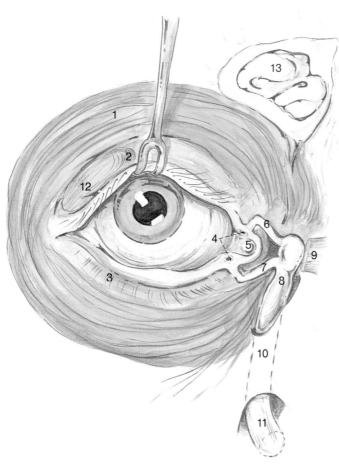

Fig. **42** Overview of the lacrimal apparatus. The eyelids have been slightly stretched; the medial palpebral ligament has been resected. The opening of the nasolacrimal duct is indicated

1 Orbicular muscle of the eye
2 Upper eyelid (anterior surface)
3 Lower eyelid (anterior surface)
4 Lacrimal points
5 Lacrimal papilla
6 Superior lacrimal duct
7 Inferior lacrimal duct
8 Lacrimal sac
9 Medial palpebral ligament
10 Nasolacrimal duct
11 Lacrimal fold
12 Lacrimal gland
13 Frontal sinus (partly opened)

Orbital Dissection

The depth of the above-mentioned space is entered with fine blunt elevators. The delicacy and vulnerability of the contiguous structures (e.g. cranial nerves, eye muscles) necessitate optical magnification under optimal illumination.

Wound Closure

Following removal or treatment of the underlying pathological process, complete hemostasis is of importance. The bipolar coagulation being applied should carefully avoid fine nerve branches. Actually, this also holds true for thicker nerve branches, such as the supraorbital branch of the trigeminal nerve, which may develop postoperative dysesthesia.

Some sutures for approximation of the orbicular eye muscle fibers may be indicated, depending on the state of tension that is present toward the end of the operation. Suction drains are placed only in exceptional cases, when there have been injuries to the frontal sinus mucosa. Fine interrupted sutures will close the skin incision.

Potential Errors and Dangers

— Cosmetically unsatisfactory incision
— Avoidable transection of the supraorbital branch of the trigeminal nerve
— Inadequate hemostasis in superficial and deep wound layers
— Avoidable damage to ocular muscles and intraorbital nerves
— Avoidable damage to the mucosa of the frontal sinus

Lateral Extracranial Approach to the Orbit (Krönlein)

Typical Indications for Surgery

— Processes in the lateral orbit
— Processes in the retrobulbar space
— Reconstruction after laterobasal orbital fractures

Principal Anatomical Structures

Auriculotemporal nerve, superficial temporal artery and vein, facial artery and vein, temporal and zygomatic branches of the facial nerve, anterior auricular muscle, orbicular muscle of the eye, epicranial muscle, temporoparietal muscle, temporal fascia, zygomatic bone (frontal and temporal processes), frontozygomatic suture, temporozygomatic suture, temporal bone (zygomatic process), sphenoid bone (greater wing); rectus lateralis, inferior and superior bulbi muscles; inferior oblique muscle of the eyeball, lacrimal gland, eyeball, optic nerve, ophthalmic artery and vein, nasociliary nerve, trochlear nerve, lacrimal nerve, frontal nerve, infraorbital branch of the trigeminal nerve, ciliary ganglion, abducens nerve.

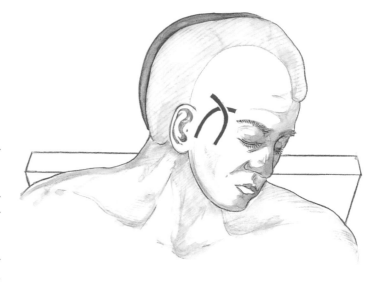

Fig. **43** Lateral extracranial approach to the orbit (Krönlein): positioning and incisions (two possible incisions)

Positioning and Skin Incision

(Fig. 43)

The patient is placed in a semisitting position, with the slightly raised head turned away from the operator by 30—35 degrees. If a particularly fine microsurgical dissection is planned, the patient's head should be rigidly restrained. The skin incision either runs from posterior-superior toward the lateral margin of the orbit and the zygomatic bone, or it takes the opposite course, that is, it curves above the lateral end of the eyebrow toward the temporal region. The latter incision usually gives better cosmetic results, but requires a somewhat larger approach. Special care should be taken to divide the skin so that the nerves and vessels of the next layer can be accessed under direct vision. The following figures show the posteriorly curved incision.

Dissection of the Superficial Temporo-Orbital Region

(Fig. 44)

The most important anatomical structures in this layer are shown in the illustration. Care is taken to identify the branches of the facial nerve in particular; these are retracted inferiorly-posteriorly as far as possible. The orbicular muscle of the eye is separated from the lateral margin of the orbit and retracted anteriorly, giving access to the fascia-invested temporal muscle.

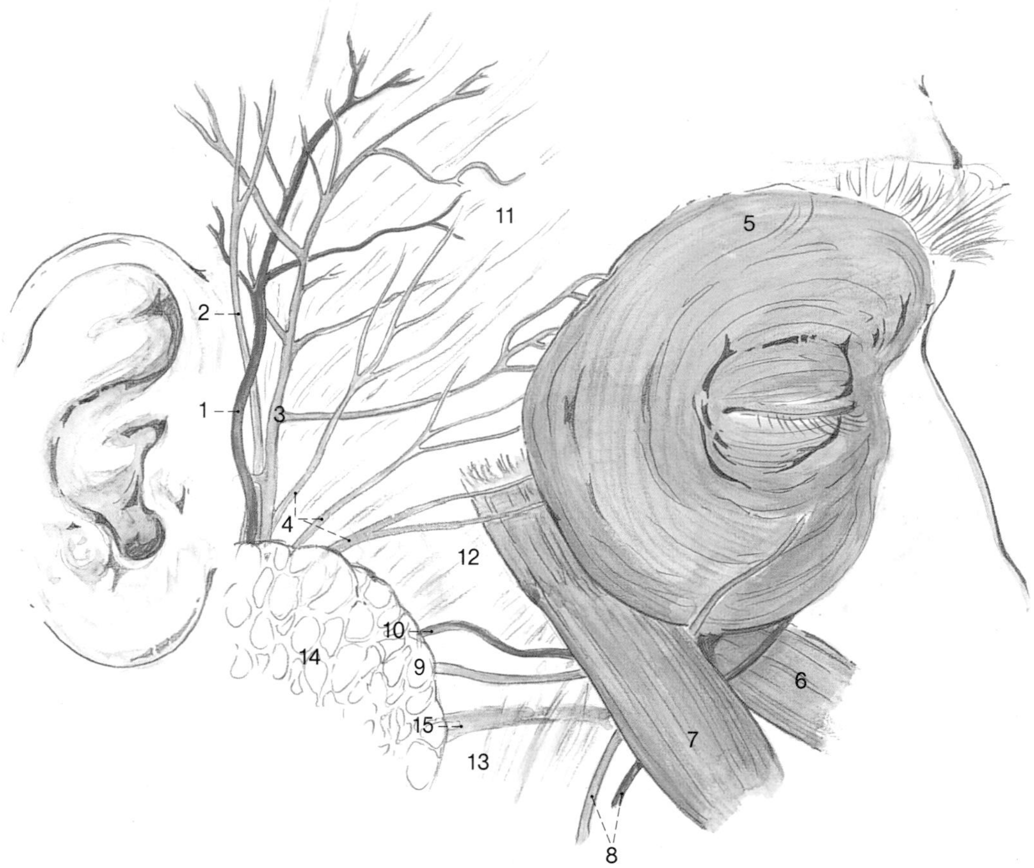

Fig. **44** The superficial anatomy of the temporal region, with nerves and vessels in their relation to the ear, eye, zygomatic arch, and parotid gland

1 Superficial temporal artery, temporal and frontal branch
2 Auriculotemporal nerve
3 Superficial temporal vein
4 Temporal and zygomatic branches of the facial nerve
5 Orbicular muscle of the eye
6 Lesser zygomatic muscle
7 Greater zygomatic muscle
8 Facial artery and vein
9 Buccal branch of the facial nerve
10 Transverse facial artery
11 Temporal fascia
12 Zygomatic arch
13 Masseteric fascia
14 Parotid gland
15 Parotid duct

Dissection of the Temporal Muscle
(Fig. **45**)

The temporal muscle is transversely incised caudally approximately one centimeter above the frontozygomatic suture, while ensuring complete hemostasis. After this, it is dissected free of the posterior border of the zygomatic bone and reflected posteriorly. An elevator is needed to retract the muscle on the sphenoid and temporal bones. The muscle is retracted from the operative field with hooks or sutures.

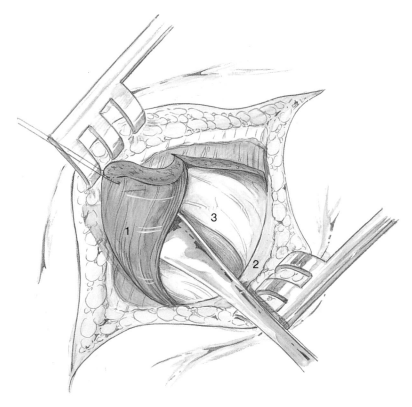

Fig. **45** Transverse incision and retraction of the temporal muscle

1 Temporal muscle
2 Zygomatic bone (frontal process)
3 Sphenoid bone (greater wing)

Resection of the Lateral Margin of the Orbit
(Fig. 46)

The next operative step is the broadest possible resection of the zygomatic bone. For this purpose, a microburr, or the Gigli saw, is used to make cuts in the border areas of the vertical portion of the zygomatic bone, that is, cranially in the vicinity of the frontozygomatic suture and caudally at the rectangular knee.

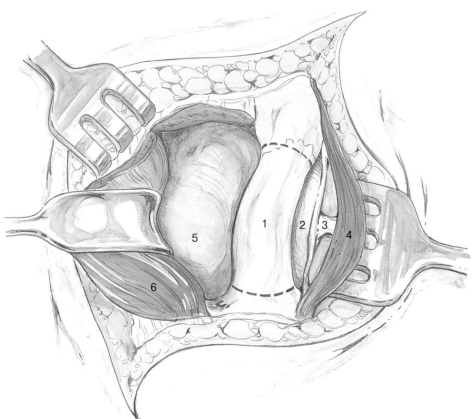

Fig. **46**   Resection of the lateral orbital border

1 Zygomatic bone (frontal process) with resection lines
2 Detached periorbita
3 Lateral palpebral ligament
4 Orbicular muscle of the eye
5 Sphenoid bone (greater wing)
6 Retracted temporal muscle

Lateral Orbitotomy
(Fig. 47)

A burr hole is placed in the anterior superior angle of the exposed lateral orbital wall, and from this burr hole the lateral wall of the orbit is removed osteoclastically with microburrs or fine punches, or both. If the local anatomical conditions are particularly favorable, including a moderately developed temporal muscle, the lateral orbital wall can also be removed osteoplastically.

In the next step, the periorbita can be incised longitudinally and transversely. This will gradually give access to the normal and pathological structures in the orbital funnel. The normal structures are shown in Figure **48**.

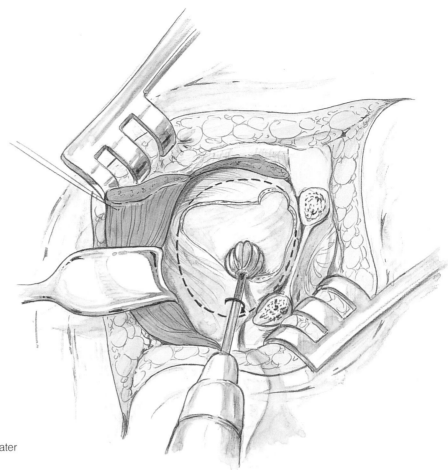

Fig. **47** Burr opening of the lateral orbital wall (greater wing of sphenoid bone). The periorbita is visualized

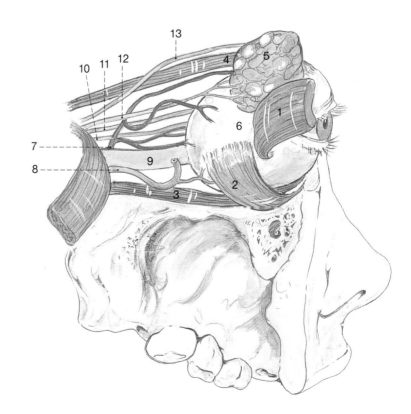

Fig. **48** Anatomy of the orbital contents; lateral view

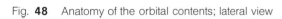

1 Rectus lateralis bulbi muscle
2 Inferior oblique muscle of the eyeball
3 Rectus inferior bulbi muscle
4 Rectus superior bulbi muscle
5 Lacrimal gland
6 Eyeball
7 Ophthalmic artery
8 Ophthalmic vein
9 Optic nerve
10 Nasociliary nerve
11 Trochlear nerve
12 Lacrimal nerve
13 Frontal nerve

● Beware: ciliary ganglion

Dissection Inside the Orbit
(Fig. 49)

All the steps in the dissection have to be carried out under optimal illumination and optical magnification so as to spare in large part the extremely vulnerable structures around the optic nerve and the eye. This has to begin with retraction of the very finely granular orbital fat, which tends to prolapse into the operative field unless use is made of slender spatulas. Further dissection in a predominantly horizontal direction leads to the muscles, vessels, and nerves, and finally reaches the targeted pathological process.

Closure of Soft-Tissue Layers
(Fig. 50)

After reexamination of the hemostasis in the operative field, closure is begun with suture of the periorbita. If the temporal portion of the bone has been preserved, it is now reimplanted, retention sutures being used to impart a degree of stability to adjacent periosteal and muscular areas. The excised lateral orbital border can be anchored much more securely at its site of removal with the aid of sutures, wire sutures, or fine plates that are passed through the bone. After this, sutures are placed between the orbicular muscle of the eye and the adjacent periosteum.

The last step consists of approximating the temporal muscle in the direction of the fibers and closing the fascia.

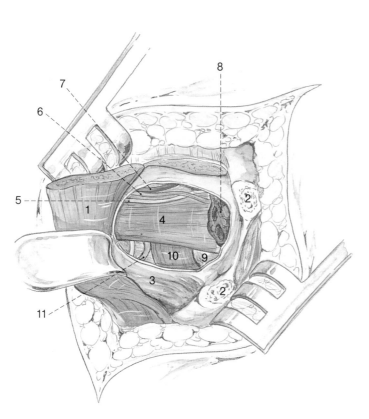

Fig. **49**   Dissection of muscles and nerves in the lateral orbit

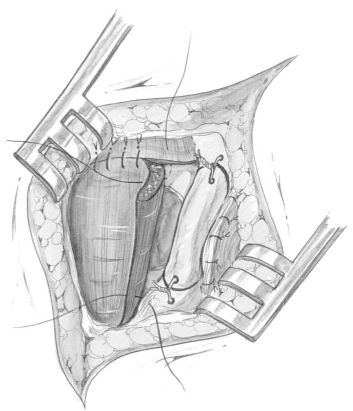

Fig. **50**   Closure of bones and musculature after lateral orbitotomy

 1 Temporal muscle
 2 Resection surfaces of frontal process of zygomatic bone
 3 Sphenoid bone (greater wing)
 4 Rectus lateralis bulbi muscle
 5 Lacrimal nerve
 6 Superior ophthalmic vein
 7 Lacrimal artery
 8 Lacrimal gland
 9 Eyeball
10 Inferior oblique muscle of eyeball
11 Inferior ophthalmic vein

Wound Closure

Once hemostasis in each layer has again been verified, a decision can be taken on whether to insert a suction drain, which is brought out posteriorly through a separate incision.

In conclusion, cosmetically treated interrupted skin sutures are applied.

Potential Errors and Dangers

— Inadequate hemostasis in the various dissection layers
— Avoidable damage to branches of the facial nerve
— Avoidable damage to intraorbital nerves and ocular muscles
— Avoidable damage to the optic nerve and the central artery of the retina
— Insufficient lateral support of the orbital contents
— Inadequate anchoring of the reimplanted lateral orbital border
— Cosmetically inadequate suture of the skin wound

3   Approaches to the Frontotemporal Junction

Unilateral Extradural Approach to the Frontotemporal Junction

Typical Indications for Surgery

— Lateral sphenoid wing meningioma
— Lateral infiltrative orbital and paranasal sinus tumors
— Localized injuries

Principal Anatomical Structures

Temporoparietal muscle, superficial temporal artery and vein, auriculotemporal nerve, zygomatic branches of the facial nerve, galea aponeurotica, temporal bone (pars squamosa), sphenoid bone (greater wing), zygomatic process of the temporal bone, middle meningeal artery, dura mater, superior ophthalmic vein, frontal bone (pars orbitalis).

Positioning and Skin Incisions

(Fig. 51)

The patient is placed in a supine position and the head is turned to the contralateral side by 30–45 degrees; this places the operative field in a nearly horizontal plane. Firm fixation may be useful, and may on occasion be necessary. Suitable skin incisions include a moderately arched local incision within the hairline as well as the so-called Unterberger incision, extending from just anterior to one ear to the beginning of the other ear; the latter is generally used for cosmetic reasons. In the areas just anterior to the ear,

special care has to be taken to avoid injury to the temporal and zygomatic branches of the facial nerve and to the auriculotemporal nerve. Division of branches of the superficial and middle temporal vein and artery can be limited, but is not avoidable; only bipolar coagulation should be used in this area.

Dissection of Soft Tissues

Once the skin flap has been retracted laterally or toward the eyebrows, and the transected cutaneous vessel branches have been securely closed by coagulation and clamps as well as Cologne clips, an arcuate incision can be made in the galea aponeurotica to permit closure by suture at the end of the operation. Now the temporal muscle can be stripped from the bone. This operative step may involve considerable bleeding and effort, particularly in the presence of sphenoid wing tumors, because these tumors are supplied with blood from the often massively dilated branches of the middle meningeal artery and the superficial temporal artery. Therefore, in preparing for this operation, it is necessary to consider preoperative embolization of these vessels, or of the tumor portions being supplied, as well as possible ligation in the area of the external carotid artery. Local hemostasis needs to be performed rapidly and with precision. Coagulation is adequate on the medial side of the muscle; wax and (rarely) impaction with a chisel are required on the bone surface. In the presence of perforating tumors, definitive hemostasis cannot be accomplished until after the completed craniotomy. The redissected temporal muscle is withdrawn from the operative field with retractors or strong traction sutures.

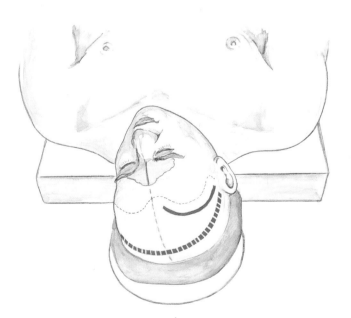

Fig. **51**   Unilateral extradural approach to the frontotemporal region: positioning and incisions. *Yellow:* frontal sinus

Craniotomy
(Fig. 52)

The number and arrangement of the burr holes depend on the size and exact location of the tumors, which are determined preoperatively mostly by detailed radiography and computed tomography. If the craniotome is used and the squamous part of the temporal bone has not been invaded by the tumor, a single burr hole, consistent with the surgeon's dexterity, is sufficient. Involvement and infiltration of the temporal bone require an osteoplastic approach via healthy bony areas and subsequent osteoclastic removal of the altered portions of bone. This step, too, tends to be associated with massive bleeding, and wax is needed to control it. Occasionally, it is also necessary to trace the middle meningeal artery in the direction of the base of the skull, where it is coagulated or tamponaded.

The bone flap is temporarily removed as a rule (packed under sterile, moist conditions). However, it may also be left in place on the muscle, depending on the extent of the localized hemorrhages.

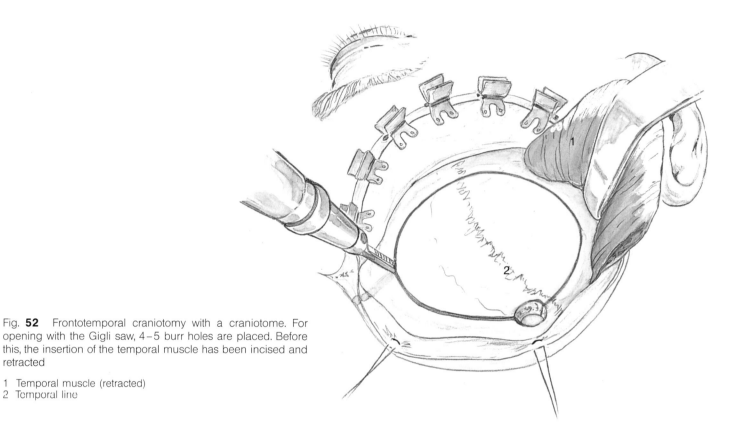

Fig. **52** Frontotemporal craniotomy with a craniotome. For opening with the Gigli saw, 4–5 burr holes are placed. Before this, the insertion of the temporal muscle has been incised and retracted

1 Temporal muscle (retracted)
2 Temporal line

Retraction of Dura-Invested Brain
(Fig. 53)

In the next step, supported by dehydrating measures by the anesthetist, the dura-invested brain is gradually, without much pressure, retracted with the aid of spatulas. This generally applies to a lateral sphenoid wing meningioma growing en plaque, and to injuries. If the dura, too, has been invaded by the tumor, it is divided at a sufficient distance from the tumor margin, and is later reconstructed. A tumor growing en plaque extends to varying degrees across the orbital and sloping portions of the lateral sphenoid wing; it may have eroded or penetrated the periosteum and reached adjacent portions of various paranasal sinuses. On the basis of anatomic preparations and computed tomograms, Figure **54** shows the sometimes very wide-ranging frontal sinuses, which can be reached by the tumor as well as by surgical dissection, and from which tumors may also originate.

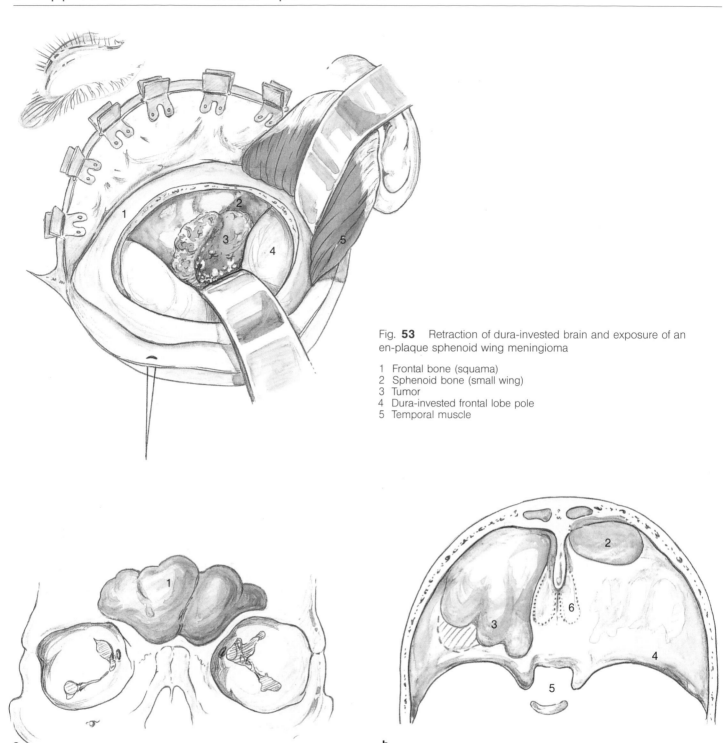

Fig. **53**   Retraction of dura-invested brain and exposure of an en-plaque sphenoid wing meningioma

1 Frontal bone (squama)
2 Sphenoid bone (small wing)
3 Tumor
4 Dura-invested frontal lobe pole
5 Temporal muscle

a   b

Fig. **54**   Possible extent of the usually asymmetrical frontal sinuses; **a** from the front; **b** from above

1 Ventral wall of the frontal sinuses after removal of the external lamina of the frontal bone
2 Average extent of the frontal sinus in the adult (hatching: possible extension)
3 Extreme extent of the frontal sinus in the adult (hatching: possible extension)
4 Sphenoid bone (small wing)
5 Hypophyseal fossa
6 Cribriform lamina

The approach in the frontotemporal area is also determined by the shape of the orbital roof, various configurations of which are shown schematically in Figure **55**, again on the basis of anatomic preparations. A highly arched orbital roof poses a problem particularly in the pterional approach, which is described below (p. 49).

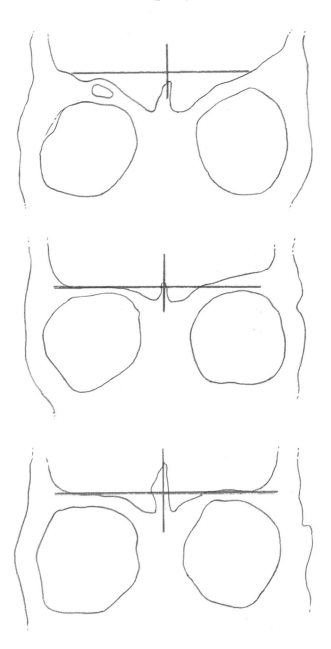

Bone and Wound Closure
(Fig. **56**)

Placement of dural elevation sutures, which are passed through the bone margin, is recommended to minimize the possibility of a postoperative epidural hematoma. This operative step can easily be added immediately after the craniotomy; it is then merely necessary to tie the sutures at the end of the operation. For fixation of the reimplanted bone flap, dural sutures passed through the bone, which are likewise tied over the flap and which additionally secure the epidural space, are recommended. A well-developed periosteum may also be used for suture.

In the next step, the temporal muscle is reflected and sutured to the galea aponeurotica. Osteoclastically removed portions of bone, which usually have a basal location, are fully covered by muscle.

A single-layer or multilayer wound closure, with careful reverification of the hemostasis, completes the operation.

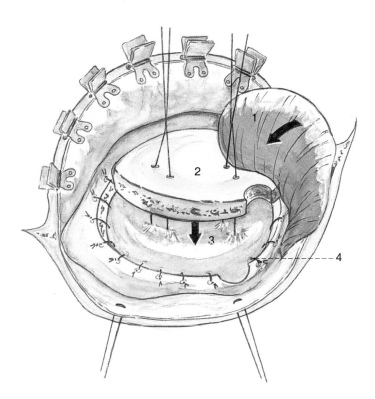

Fig. **55** Variations in shape and course of the orbital roof, based on anatomical preparations. This greatly diminishes the surgeon's view of the paramedian and median structures at the base of the brain (e.g., branches of the anterior cerebral artery). The red lines adjoin the lateral osseous site of reflection, as well as the middle of the bony base of the skull

Fig. **56** Closure of the frontotemporal craniotomy and wound

1 Temporal muscle
2 Bone flap with central dural elevation sutures
3 Dura mater
4 Circular dural elevation sutures (passed through the bone)

Potential Errors and Dangers

– Injury to major branches of the facial nerve
– Underestimated blood loss due to inadequate hemostasis
– Overlooked and therefore untreated development of communication with the paranasal sinuses, with associated risk of infection

– Unintended, but often unavoidable, injury to the dura during preparation of the bone flap by saw or burr owing to strong adhesions between the dura and the internal periosteal layer, or to tumor infiltration
– Postoperative epidural hematoma due to inadequate or excessively slack dural elevation sutures
– Soft-tissue hematoma

Unilateral Intradural Approach to the Frontotemporal Junction

Typical Indications for Surgery

— Processes in the sella-chiasma region
— Selected aneurysms
— Intradural sphenoid wing tumors
— Intradural and extradural sphenoid wing tumors

Principal Anatomical Structures

Temporoparietal muscle, superficial temporal artery and vein, auriculotemporal nerve, zygomatic branches of the facial nerve, galea aponeurotica, temporal bone (pars squamosa), sphenoid bone (greater wing), zygomatic process of the temporal bone, middle meningeal artery, dura mater, superior ophthalmic vein, maxillary nerve, ophthalmic nerve, oculomotor nerve, olfactory nerve and bulb, optic nerve and optic chiasm, internal carotid artery (pars cavernosa and pars cerebri), ophthalmic artery, cavernous sinus, abducens nerve, pituitary gland, hypophyseal stalk, diaphragm of the sella turcica, crista galli.

Positioning and Skin Incision

(Fig. **57**)

The patient is in supine position with the head turned to the opposite side (usually left) by 30–45 degrees. If required by

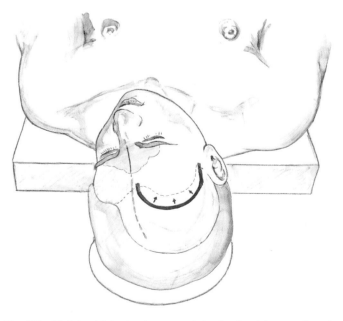

Fig. **57** Unilateral intradural approach to the frontotemporal region: positioning and incision. *Yellow:* frontal sinuses; *black arrows:* hairline

the intricacy of the planned procedure, the head is fixed using three-point skull fixation.

The typical skin incision describes an arc – the size of which is determined by the target object – within the frontotemporal hairline. On occasion, cosmetic considerations require a bow-shaped incision, extending from the border of one ear to the other.

Anteriorly to the anterior upper border of the ear, particular attention has to be paid to the temporal and zygomatic branches of the facial nerve and to the auriculotemporal nerve.

Branches of the superficial temporal artery and vein cannot always be bypassed; they are subjected to bipolar coagulation.

Dissection of Soft Tissues

When the skin flap has been retracted toward its base with the aid of shallow passage of a scalpel and, in part, with a pledget, hemorrhages should be controlled by bipolar coagulation, and the margins of the incision closed with clamps or clips. Elevation sutures or a transposable fishhook keep the skin flap permanently out of the operative field. An arcuate incision is made in the galea aponeurotica at a distance of one centimeter from the tendinous portion of the temporal muscle; the muscle is subsequently retracted from its support, and the fishhook is applied at a different site, or another elevation suture is passed through the muscle base. During dissection in these basal regions, particular attention should be paid to the exposed vessels and nerves, shown in Figure **58**. The relations between nerves and vessels vary individually; thus, the auriculotemporal nerve not infrequently passes through the loop of the superficial temporal artery.

Craniotomy

To open the bone, use can be made of several burr holes that are subsequently joined with the Gigli saw or a craniotome; or a single burr hole can be placed, depending on the operator's dexterity. The size of the craniotomy is determined by the surgeon according to the target process and to his own views; one should aim for the smallest possible craniotomy without compromising access. Hemorrhages occurring during the craniotomy, particularly in the case of infiltrative tumors, call for rapid surgery so that local hemorrhages can then be controlled by bipolar and monopolar coagulation and wax.

The bone flap may either be temporarily removed or left in place on the muscle. Here again, careful hemostasis is required prior to further operative steps. For optimal utilization of the approach opening, the fishhook is attached, or a muscle elevation suture is passed over the bone flap.

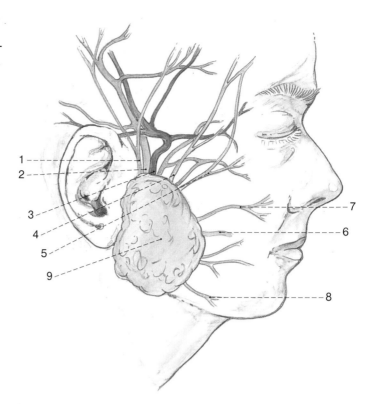

Fig. **58** Anatomy of the right-sided superficial temporal region. The order of succession of the nerve and vessel trunks varies considerably

1 Auriculotemporal nerve
2 Superficial temporal vein
3 Superficial temporal artery
4 Temporal branches of the facial nerve
5 Zygomatic branches of the facial nerve
6 Parotid duct
7 Buccal branches of the facial nerve
8 Marginal mandibular branch of the facial nerve
9 Parotid gland

Opening the Dura
(Fig. **59**)

Placement of dural elevation sutures, which are drawn into channels drilled through the bone margin and are not at first tied, is recommended before the actual incision of the dura. The sutures are tied toward the end of the operation, that is, after closure of the dural opening, so that no irreversible traction on the dural borders is produced. The arcuate incision is given a central base, and is kept at a distance of several millimeters from the bone margin so as not to hamper the final dural suture. For full utilization of the craniotomy, tangential incisions in the direction of the bone margin are added.

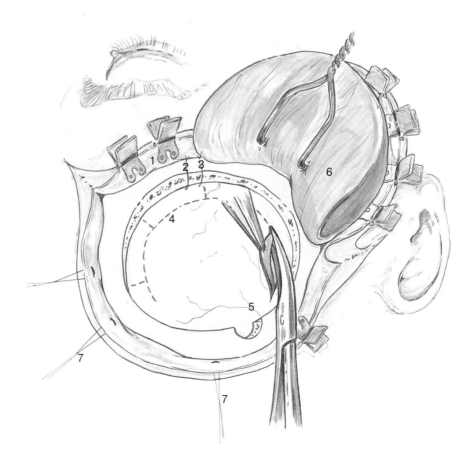

Fig. **59** The craniotome-cut bone flap has been removed. The dura mater is incised along the dashed red line

1 Galea aponeurotica
2 Frontal bone (squama)
3 Dural elevation sutures (passed through the bone)
4 Dura mater with dural incision line
5 Branches of the middle meningeal artery
6 Temporal muscle (reflected superiorly)
7 Galeal elevation sutures

Development of the Chiasmal Region
(Fig. **60**)

Elevation sutures through the dural flaps provide for an optimal opening. Now, at the latest, the operating microscope should be used. The frontal flap can be raised and displaced medially, generally with the use of a self-retaining spatula, supported by the anesthetist's dehydrating measures. Alongside the border of the sphenoid wing, and anteriorly to the temporal pole, the cisterna carotidea is encountered and, a small distance inward from it, the internal carotid artery and the immediately adjacent optic nerve. Adjoining it is the dura-invested portion of the orbital roof. A thin cottonoid strip can be placed under the spatula; natural protection is also afforded by leaving the circumcised dural flap in place. The other adjacent structures are brought into the field of vision by modified spatula maneuvers in conjunction with adjusted viewing angles. A semidiagrammatic representation of a typical viewing angle is provided in Figure **61**, without, however, showing the overlying brain and with the anterior cerebral arteries and the anterior communicating artery displaced posteriorly. The diaphragma sellae and emerging tumors are seen in the brown area of the drawing. The approach may also require dissection between the optic nerve and the internal carotid artery. For aneurysms of the internal carotid artery and its adjacent branches, the pterional approach, described in the following chapter, is preferred. The same applies to retrosellar processes. The individual anatomical situation of the optic chiasm, that is, its anterior or posterior position, influences any procedure in the anterior chiasmatic angle. The posterior position naturally facilitates this approach. In the anterior position, portions of the posterior border of the sellar tubercle may have to be removed with a burr in order to achieve the necessary approach.

After completion of the intradural procedure, the dural incision is closed; interrupted or continuous sutures may be employed for this purpose. If tension has developed in the dural plane, or if a fragment of the dura has been resected, or if several small gaps remain in the dura, implantation or coverage with a plastic material is required; this in turn is then sutured or glued, or both.

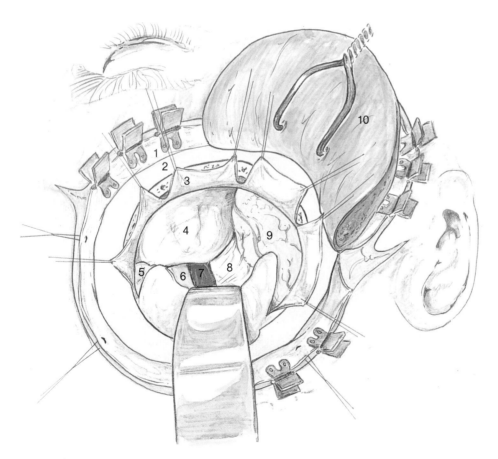

Fig. **60**   Clarification of the chiasmatic region

1 Galea aponeurotica
2 Frontal bone (squama)
3 Dura mater (incised)
4 Frontal bone (orbital part)
5 Frontal lobe
6 Right optic nerve
7 Right internal carotid artery
8 Carotid cistern
9 Pole of the temporal lobe
10 Temporal muscle (folded back)

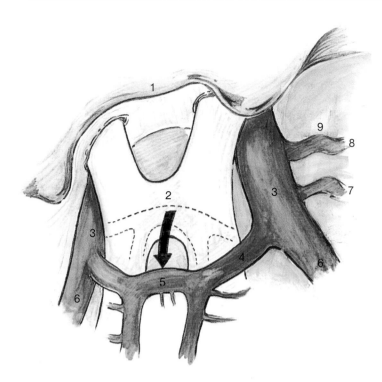

Bone and Wound Closure
(Fig. **62**)

In the next step, dural elevation sutures extending around the circumference of the bone opening are inserted, or elevation sutures are inserted and tied after the bone flap has been replaced, so as to minimize the chance of a space-occupying postoperative epidural hematoma developing. The bone flap can be readily fixed with dural elevation sutures that are likewise passed through the central bone. To this are added sutures between the temporal muscle, which has been reflected to its original position, and the galea aponeurotica, transverse tension sutures possibly being used for reinforcement.

After final verification of hemostasis and the occasionally required insertion of a suction drain, a single-layer wound closure can be carried out with interrupted sutures. The operation is completed by fixation of a drain with the aid of an interrupted suture.

Fig. **61**   The schematic anatomy of the sella-chiasm region. The anterior communicating artery has been retracted posteriorly. Its actual situation is identified by black shading

1 Sphenoidal jugum
2 Left and right optic nerve, optic chiasm, and optic tract
3 Left and right internal carotid artery
4 Right anterior cerebral artery
5 Anterior communicating artery
6 Left and right middle cerebral artery
7 Right anterior choroidal artery
8 Right posterior communicating artery

Fig. **62**   Reinsertion of the bone flap and wound closure

1 Temporal muscle
2 Bone flap with central dural elevation sutures
3 Dura mater, closed with continuous and interrupted sutures
4 Circular dural elevation sutures (passed through the bone)

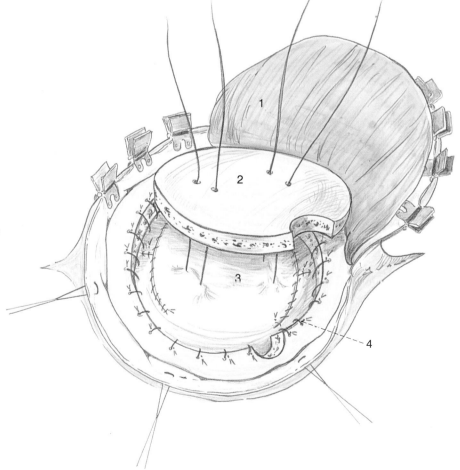

Potential Errors and Dangers

— Injury to heavier branches of the facial nerve during the skin incision
— Overlooked loss of blood due to inadequate hemostasis at the cutaneous level
— Overlooked, but often unavoidable, injury to the dura during preparation of the bone flap with the use of a saw or craniotome, owing to firm adhesions between the dura and the internal periosteum
— Injuries to the numerous nerves and vessels in the chiasma region
— Injuries to adjacent portions of the frontal and temporal lobes due to spatula pressure
— Postoperative epidural hematoma due to inadequate or slack dural elevation sutures
— Soft-tissue hematoma

Pterional Intradural Approach to the Frontotemporal Junction

This approach was designed and fully developed by M.G. Yaşargil. It is described below in accordance with his directions.

Typical Indications for Surgery

- Aneurysms of the internal carotid artery and its branches
- Aneurysms of the superior portions of the basilar artery and its branches
- Tumors in the superior, posterior, and lateral orbital regions
- Tumors within, above, and behind the sella
- Tumors of the optic chiasm and adjoining portions of the optic nerve
- Tumors above, on the side of, behind, and in front of the optic chiasm
- Tumors in the area of the clivus
- Tumors anterior to the pons
- Scars secondary to inflammations in the chiasm-optic nerve region

Principal Anatomical Structures

Temporoparietal muscle, superficial temporal artery and vein, auriculotemporal nerve, zygomatic branches of the facial nerve, galea aponeurotica, frontal bone (squama and pars orbitalis), sphenoid bone (greater and lesser wings), zygomatic process of frontal bone, parietal bone (sphenoid angle), coronal suture, sphenosquamous suture, zygomatic process of temporal bone, middle meningeal artery, dura mater, superior ophthalmic vein, maxillary nerve, ophthalmic nerve, oculomotor nerve, olfactory nerve, subarachnoidal supratentorial cisterns, optic nerve and optic chiasm, internal carotid artery (cavernous and cerebral parts) and its branches, with transition to the basilar artery, cavernous sinus, abducens nerve, pituitary and hypophyseal stalk, diaphragm of the sella turcica, veins of the base and the dorsal brain stem.

Positioning and Skin Incision

(Fig. **63**)

The patient is placed in a supine position. As the positioning has to be very exact and needs to be steadily maintained (surgical microscope), the patient's head should be fixed in a three-pin head clamp that is firmly connected to the oper-

ating table. The single pin is placed on the side of the operation, behind the ear and above the mastoid, while the double pins are placed on the contralateral side at the frontotemporal junction and above the temporal line (outside the temporal muscle).

For the (mostly right-sided) craniotomy, the patient's head is tilted backward by 20 degrees, slightly raised at the neck, and turned 30–35 degrees to the left. The desired central reference point is the frontozygomatic suture; the operator should have a direct topside view of it in both planes. Any rotation and tilting of the head requires the anesthetist's cooperation so that respiration and blood flow are not compromised.

The arcuate incision starts 2–3 cm to the side of the midline within the hairline, and extends to a point just short of the anterior superior border of the ear. In order to spare the trunk of the superficial temporal artery, it is marked beforehand.

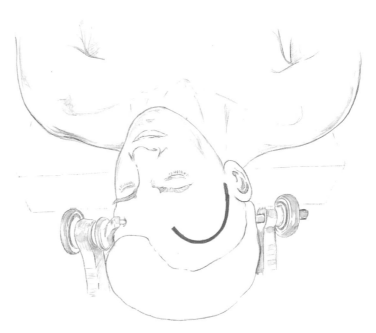

Fig. **63** Pterional approach to the frontotemporal base of the skull: positioning and incision

Dissection of Soft Tissues
(Fig. 64)

The skin flap is dissected from the superficial fascia of the temporal muscle by shallow advance of the scalpel blade and with the use of small, firm pledgets, and it is retracted with fishhooks. This is followed by arcuate incisions through the fascia and periosteum, as shown in the illustration. After this, the frontal periosteal flap is reflected anteriorly, and the flap facing the longitudinal sinus is reflected toward the surgeon. At the base of the operative field, the two layers of the superficial temporal fascia are transected (dashed line). A small artery emerging from the bone at the anterior border, and a larger, obliquely running vein closer to the temporal region, require bipolar coagulation (Fig. 65).

At the boundary of the frontal process of the zygomatic bone, an incision is made along the border of the temporal muscle so that the muscle can then be freed from the bone step by step. Thus, the direction of the dissection is posterior-inferior; the muscle is removed from the operative field for a commensurate distance, and temporal branches of the facial nerve are spared to a large extent. The next layer is kept out of the field of vision by means of fishhooks or additional elevation sutures.

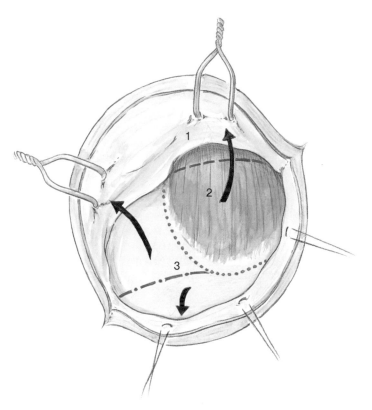

Fig. **64** Incision of the fascia and periosteum. *Dashed line:* transection of temporal muscle; *dotted line:* fascial-periosteal incision near the temporal line; *dash-dot line:* periosteal incision on the squama of the frontal bone diagonally to the medial wound margin

1 Galea aponeurotica
2 Temporal muscle, covered with fascia
3 Periosteum of frontal bone squama

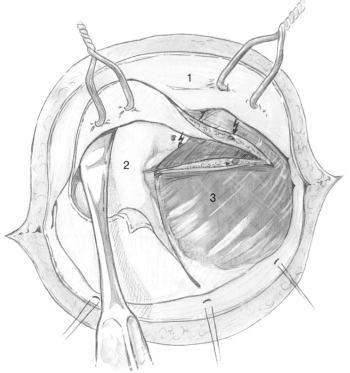

Fig. **65** Dissection of the fascia and transverse incision of the temporal muscle

1 Galea aponeurotica
2 Frontal bone (squama)
3 Temporal muscle with divided and coagulated local artery and vein

Craniotomy
(Fig. 66)

In the bony area thus exposed, the drill holes are to be placed in a pattern that is identified in the figure by capital letters. The first burr hole (A) is placed directly inward from the temporal line immediately above the frontozygomatic suture; this is followed by a frontal hole (B) 2 cm above the orbital margin and outside the frontal sinus in the frontal bone. The third hole (C) lies in the parietal bone behind the coronal suture on the temporal line, and the fourth hole (D)

is placed in the squama of the temporal bone behind the sphenosquamous suture. The holes are joined with the craniotome or Gigli saw. To avoid dural injuries, the dura is retracted as far as possible with Braatz probes before drilling, particularly so between burr holes A and B.

Starting from drill hole A, a wide microburr is used to cut a channel in the direction of hole D; this channel thus forms the boundary of the bone flap and allows the craniotomy to be carried as far as the temporal base. During the subsequent operation, the removed bone flap is packed off under sterile and moist conditions. Additional space can be created at the base with the aid of Luer forceps of various sizes and shapes, punches, and a liquid-cooled burr. This affects the lateral sphenoid wing (Fig. **67**) and adjoining high-domed portions of the orbital roof. Prior to these mea-

sures, one to two small incisions are made in the exposed dura to allow cerebrospinal fluid to drip off (Fig. **67**). This operative step should provide a pyramid-shaped view toward the sella that is not obstructed by basal bony structures.

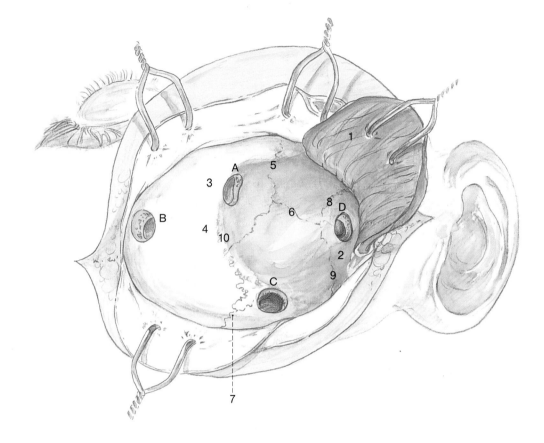

Fig. **66** Localization of burr holes (letters mark the order of succession)

1 Temporal muscle (reflected)
2 Sphenoid bone (great wing)
3 Zygomatic bone (frontal process)
4 Frontal bone (zygomatic process)
5 Frontozygomatic suture
6 Sphenofrontal suture
7 Coronal suture
8 Sphenosquamous suture
9 Squamous suture
10 Superior temporal line

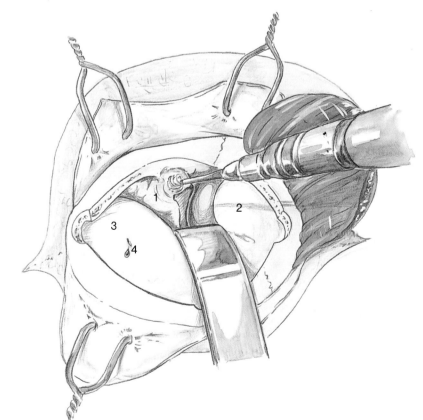

Fig. **67** Retraction of dura-invested brain, small dural incision for cerebrospinal fluid outflow, and ablation of high-rising portions of the sphenoid wing and adjacent parts of the orbital roof

1 Sphenoid bone (small wing)
2 Dura-covered pole of the temporal lobe
3 Dura-covered portion of the frontal lobe
4 Incision in the dura mater for drop-by-drop drainage of cerebrospinal fluid

Opening the Dura
(Fig. 68)

The preferred next step is drilling of the bone for the dural elevation sutures; these sutures are then placed, but are not tied. After this, the usual arcuate opening with an anterior-inferior stalk can be made in the dura. The incision to an extent surrounds the base of the sylvian fossa. The resulting dural flap is reflected toward the base and fixed. Bipolar closure of the dural vessels is required only occasionally. Slight elevation of the lateral frontal lobe visualizes the cisterns in the area of the optic nerve, the internal carotid artery, and the optic chiasm. Escaping cerebrospinal fluid has to be drained for varying periods.

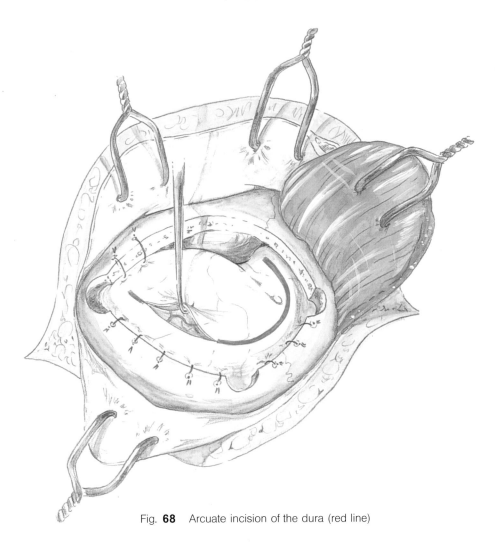

Fig. **68** Arcuate incision of the dura (red line)

Dissection of the Lateral Sulcus (Sylvian Fossa)
(Fig. 69)

Opening the cisterns causes additional cerebrospinal fluid to run out, so that the pyramid-shaped view is gradually widened more and more. Under normal circumstances, a sequence of steps is observed that is essentially determined by the location of the pathologic process, but generally begins with the carotid and interpeduncular cisterns. This is followed, as a rule, by dissection of the cistern of the Sylvian fossa along the large sulcus lateralis vein. This essentially opens the way to the approach to the internal carotid artery and its branches; it needs to be enlarged in keeping with the area being targeted. The general situation of the cisterns in this region is shown in Figure **70**; the field of vision resulting is presented in Figure **71**.

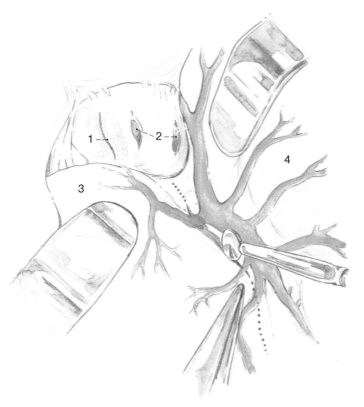

Fig. **69**   Dissection of the lateral fissure alongside the superficial middle cerebral vein, and opening of the carotid and interpeduncular cisterns

1   Incision over the carotid cistern
2   Incisions over the interpeduncular cistern
3   Frontal lobe
4   Temporal lobe

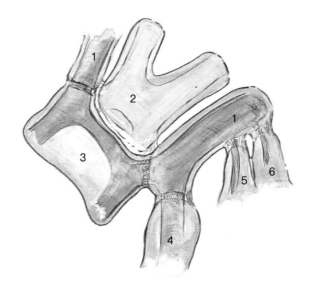

Fig. **70**   The subarachnoid spaces in the chiasmatic region (Yaşargil 1984)

1   Carotid cistern
2   Chiasmatic cistern
3   Cistern of terminal lamina
4   Cistern of lateral fossa of cerebrum
5   Ambient cistern
6   Interpeduncular cistern

Dura, Bone, and Wound Closure

The dura is closed with interrupted or continuous sutures, the latter requiring intermittent knots. Next, the dural elevation sutures are tied. The reimplanted bone flap can be secured with transosseous dural elevation sutures. The operation is completed with sutures of the muscle, fascia, and skin.

Potential Errors and Dangers

— Overlooked loss of blood due to inadequate hemostasis at the cutaneous level
— Dural injuries caused by the craniotome or saw; these are usually unavoidable because of existing adhesions to the bone
— Injuries to the numerous nerves and vessels
— Injuries to adjacent brain regions due to spatula pressure
— Postoperative epidural hematoma due to inadequate or slack dural elevation sutures
— Soft-tissue hematoma

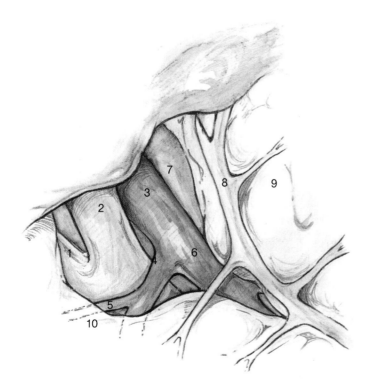

Fig. **71**   The site of the carotid artery division after removal of the arachnoid

1   Left optic nerve
2   Right optic nerve
3   Right internal carotid artery
4   Right anterior cerebral artery
5   Anterior communicating artery
6   Right middle cerebral artery
7   Oculomotor nerve
8   Superficial middle cerebral vein
9   Temporal lobe
10   Frontal lobe

4 Approaches in the Area of the Middle Cranial Fossa

Intradural Approach to the Middle Cranial Fossa

Typical Indications for Surgery

- Aneurysms of the posterior vasculature
- Tumors in the area of the tentorial notch
- Processes in the temporal lobe (tumors, arteriovenous malformations, inflammatory processes, malformations, traumas)
- Clival tumors
- Cavernous sinus processes
- Surgery for epilepsy

Principal Anatomical Structures

Superficial temporal artery and vein, temporoparietal muscle, zygomatic bone, auriculotemporal nerve, zygomatic branches of the facial nerve, middle meningeal artery and vein (frontal and parietal branches), dura mater, superficial middle cerebral veins, middle cerebral artery (temporal branches), inferior anastomotic vein (Labbé's vein), temporal lobe, tentorial border, superior petrosal sinus, sphenoparietal sinus, branches of the petrosal vein, trochlear nerve, brain stem.

Positioning and Skin Incisions

(Fig. 72)

The patient is placed in a supine position, and the ipsilateral shoulder is appreciably raised. The patient's head is turned to the opposite side and is firmly fixed. The zygomatic bone should be the highest point within the operative field; this can usually be achieved by slight tilting of the head. During positioning, great care should be taken to avoid overextension of the cervical spine and associated constriction of the cervical vessels. The anesthetist, too, will specify the limits to which the head can be turned.

Frequently, a straight, vertical skin incision proves sufficient, particularly for the subtemporal approach to the tentorial notch, the basilar artery and its branches, and the lateral brain stem.

An S-shaped skin incision is chosen if extensive parts of the temporal lobe are to be exposed.

The vertical incision should, insofar as possible, spare the superficial temporal artery so as not to compromise perfusion of the skin flap and an external-internal anastomosis

that may become necessary later. The temporal muscle is divided about 2–3 cm basal to its attachment at the cranial bone; it is divided transversely to secure its final suture. Occasionally, vertical division of the temporal muscle proves sufficient; the pressure of the retractor blades on the muscular tissue then has to be kept within limits.

In the S-shaped incision, which runs in a curve to a point behind the ear and as far as the zygomatic bone, it is generally possible to reflect the bone flap together with the muscle, so that the muscle is dissected along the course of the craniotomy line.

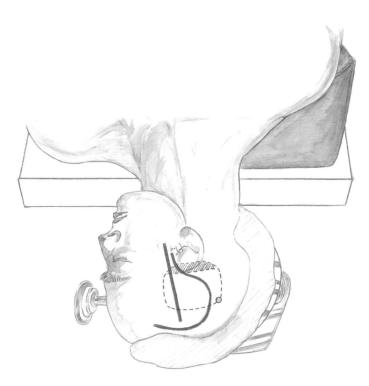

Fig. **72** Intradural approach to the middle cranial fossa: positioning and incisions (vertical incision, S-shaped incision). The bone flap to be prepared is identified by a dashed black line, and the basal portion, which is to be removed osteoclastically, by black shading. In what follows, the vertical incision is presented

Craniotomy

After the vertical skin incision, a burr hole is placed near the ear, and the craniotome is used to cut around the bone flap; an osteoclastic enlargement is required in the direction of the base. The closer this enlargement comes to the base, the easier the development of the tentorial border.

With the S-shaped skin incision, burr holes are placed at the level of the ear, and at the same level temporofrontally at the border of the temporal muscle, and an oblique cut with the craniotome is made around the bone flap. Depending on the location of the process in and near the temporal lobe, the craniotomy can be carried out more frontally toward the temporal pole, or more posteriorly toward the inferior anastomotic vein (Labbé's vein). The bone flap is broken out, the break lines are straightened and, as far as necessary, bleeding from the edges and the inside of the bone flap is stopped with bone wax. This should prevent hemorrhages from the bone flap that originate in the muscle. The bone flap is packed off wet and retracted together with the temporal muscle.

Opening the Dura
(Fig. 73)

In the vertical skin incision, the dura, for the purpose of subtemporal exposure, is opened about 2 cm parietally parallel to the base, and is then incised with scissors frontobasally and temporobasally and elevation-sutured. In the temporoparietal region, a small, folding door-like incision is made in the dura, and the resulting dural flap is used to cover the receding temporal brain. Now the effect of the downward-tilting, fixed head makes itself felt. Additional spatula pressure on the temporal brain can be kept very low without reducing the visibility of the tentorial border.

Following the S-shaped incision, an H-shaped opening can be made in the dura; its lower portion is retracted basally by suture, while the upper portion, selected according to the localization of the targeted process, has to be reflected in the parietal direction. This permits exposure of both the anterior and the posterior portions of the temporal lobe.

Figure 74 gives an overview of the structures, and especially the openings, of the middle base of the skull; the caption identifies the structures passing through.

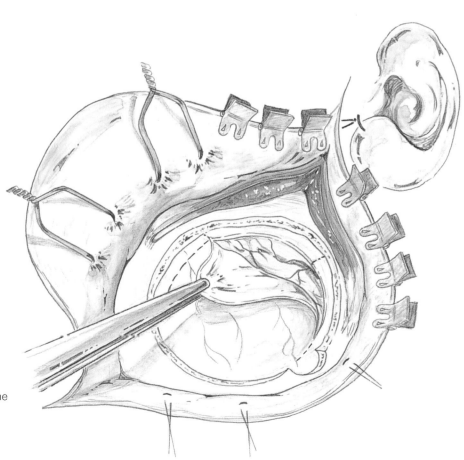

Fig. 73 The bone flap has been removed, and the basal portions of bone have been ablated osteoclastically. An arcuate incision is made around the dura along the dashed line

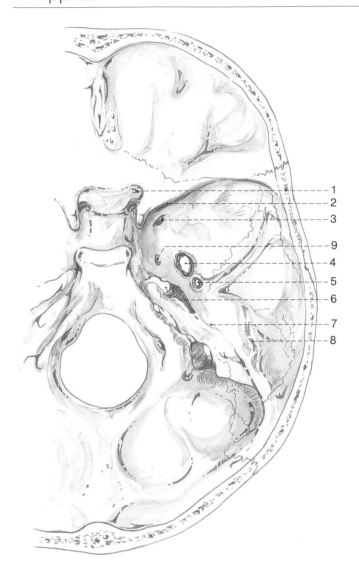

Fig. **74** The openings of the middle cranial fossa and the structures passing through it

1 Optic canal (optic nerve, ophthalmic artery)
2 Superior orbital fissure (nasociliary nerve, oculomotor nerve, abducens nerve, trochlear nerve, frontal nerve, lacrimal nerve, superior ophthalmic vein)
3 Foramen rotundum (maxillary nerve)
4 Oval foramen (mandibular nerve surrounded by the venous plexus coursing from the cavernous sinus to the pterygoid plexus)
5 Spinous foramen (middle meningeal artery, venous plexus, meningeal branch of the mandibular nerve)
6 Internal aperture of the carotid canal (internal carotid artery, internal carotid and autonomic plexus)
7 Hiatus of the canal for the greater and lesser petrosal nerve (greater and lesser petrosal nerve, superior tympanic artery)
8 Bone sulci of the middle meningeal artery
9 Venous foramen (Vesalius)

Dissection of the Middle Base of the Skull and of the Tentorial Border
(Fig. 75)

The tentorial notch is usually exposed after elevation and retraction of the temporal brain. However, if the brain pressure cannot be sufficiently modified, basal portions of the temporal lobe may have to be resected. All retracting and elevating maneuvers have to be performed slowly, cautiously, and gradually. If absolutely necessary, bridging veins should be bipolarly coagulated and divided close to the brain and far from the dura. If a sinus should be reached nonetheless, bleeding control is hampered, and tamponade and fibrin sealant may be required in some cases. Immediately adjacent to the inferior tentorial border is the trochlear nerve.

Dissection of the Temporal Lobe
(Fig. 76)

The desired resection lines of the inferior and middle temporal gyri are shown in the illustration. They are used both in epilepsy surgery and for removal of processes within the temporal lobe. The inferior anastomotic vein (Labbé's vein), situated at the parieto-occipital border, is not crossed, and should generally be spared to avoid infarctions. If it does need to be divided, a site sufficiently far from the veins and sinuses of the cranial base is chosen.

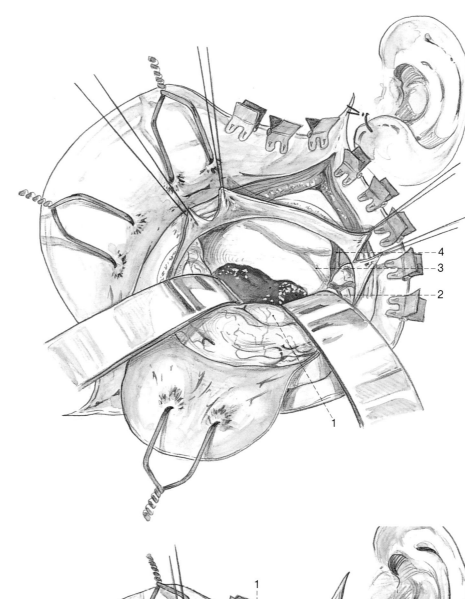

Fig. **75** The dura has been reflected, and the temporal lobe is elevated in its basal portion, visualizing the tumor

1 Inferior gyrus of temporal lobe
2 Tumor
3 Middle meningeal artery (covered by dura)
4 Inferior anastomotic vein (Labbé's vein)

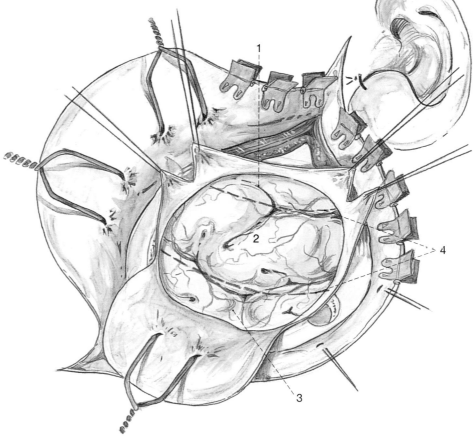

Fig. **76** Resection lines (red dashes) for the lower and middle temporal gyri

1 Inferior temporal gyrus
2 Middle temporal gyrus
3 Superior temporal gyrus
4 Resection lines

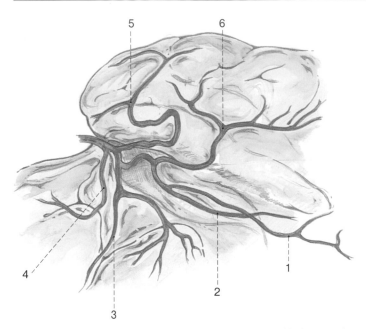

Deep within the incised temporal lobe, the branches of the middle cerebral artery are reached; their distribution is shown in Figure 77.

A caudal expansion of the approach clears the way toward and across the tentorium (Fig. 78).

Fig. **77**   The branches of the middle cerebral artery, with the lateral sulcus opened (surgical positioning)

1   Posterior temporal branch
2   Branch of angular gyri
3   Lateral frontobasal branch
4   Middle frontobasal branch
5   Anterior temporal branch
6   Intermediate temporal branch

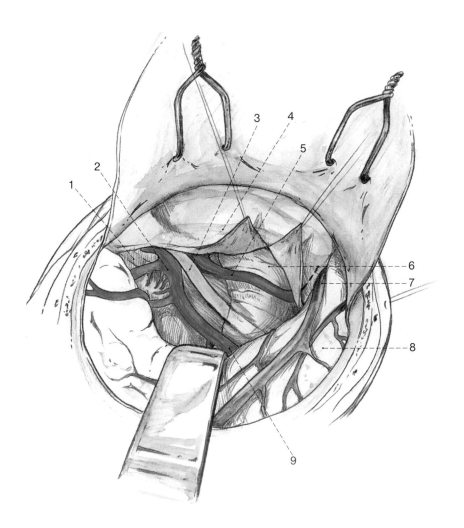

Fig. **78**   Posterior enlargement of the approach for the subtemporal route to and through the tentorium

1   Oculomotor nerve
2   Ramification of the basilar artery
3   Trochlear nerve
4   Superior petrosal sinus
5   Superior cerebellar artery
6   Cerebellum
7   Inferior anastomotic vein (Labbé's vein)
8   Temporal lobe
9   Posterior cerebral artery

Wound Closure

The dura is as a rule closed with interrupted sutures. Dural elevation sutures have to be placed with special care. The purpose, to prevent postoperative epidural hematomas, is also served by central dural elevation sutures that are passed through the bone flap. The bone flap, which usually remains at the muscle, is fitted into the craniotomy, with oblique edges facilitating the seating of the flap; it may also be connected to the cranial bone at several points on its border via small burr holes and nonabsorbable suture material.

For closure of the temporal muscle, use is made of absorbable suture material, the sutures being tied under moderate traction. The fascia of the temporal muscle is approximated with absorbable material.

Following insertion of a subcutaneous suction drain, the subcutis is sutured with absorbable material at several points. Staples or clips, as well als nonabsorbable sutures, are suitable for closure of the skin.

Potential Errors and Dangers

— Overlooked blood loss during the operation due to inadequate hemostasis of the skin flap and its cut border
— Injury of dura or cerebral cortex, or both, due to craniotomy instruments
— Pressure lesions of the brain due to improper or hasty application of brain spatulas
— Injury to the inferior anastomotic vein (Labbé's vein)
— Injury to the sphenoparietal and superior petrosal sinuses and veins entering them
— Postoperative hemorrhages due to inadequately secured vessels of the brain surface or bridging veins
— Postoperative epidural hematomas due to insufficient or slack dural elevation sutures
— Soft-tissue hematomas

Extradural Approach to the Middle Cranial Fossa

Typical Indications for Surgery

– Tumors of the trigeminal nerve
– Tumors of the extradural middle base of the skull

Principal Anatomical Structures

Superficial temporal artery and vein, auriculotemporal nerve, temporoparietal muscle, zygomatic bone, zygomatic branches of the facial nerve, middle meningeal artery and vein (frontal and parietal branches), dura mater, sphenoparietal sinus, superior petrosal sinus, cavernous sinus, middle cerebral vein, petrosal vein.

Positioning and Skin Incisions
(Fig. 79)

The patient is in a supine position; the ipsilateral shoulder is raised substantially. This allows the head to be turned in a horizontal plane without compromising the trachea or cervical vessels. In view of the delicate conditions in the operative field, the head is usually firmly fixed.

The skin may be incised either vertically or in an S-shape. The further the operative field may be expected to extend toward the cranial poles, the greater the preference for the S-shaped incision.

In the S-shaped incision, the temporal muscle is transversely notched in its upper third, so that enough muscular mass for the final muscle suture will remain on the skull. If technically feasible, the superficial temporal artery should not be divided, at least not in the trunk. Muscle retractors being used should be opened only to a moderate degree, to avoid necroses in the musculature.

Craniotomy

In the extradural procedure in particular, importance is attached to performing the craniotomy as close to the base as possible. After a burr hole has been placed, the bone flap is reamed out with slanting edges; the craniotomy defect is osteoclastically expanded toward the temporal base. In most cases, the bone flap may remain on the temporal muscle and is retracted with it.

Dissection Above the Dura Mater
(Fig. 80)

Using a fairly wide elevator, the dura on the base of the middle cranial fossa is detached in small steps. Hemorrhages, which occur very often, are controlled with bone wax, tamponade, and hemostatic fabrics. Extensive meningiomas are sometimes accessed only after resection of the investing dura mater, so that a combined procedure with the intradural approach becomes necessary in such cases. In the case of tumors of the trigeminal nerve, particularly in the area of the trigeminal cavity (Meckel's cavity), special attention has to be paid to the sphenoparietal sinus; controlling it may prove very difficult and time-consuming.

Information on the anatomical structures of the middle cranial base is provided in Figures 74 and 81.

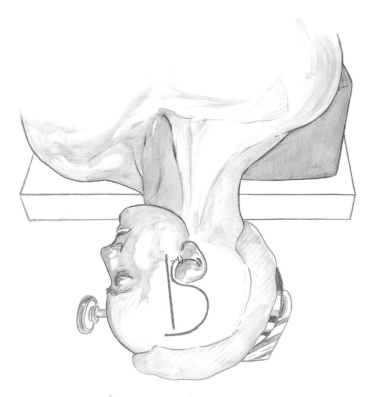

Fig. 79   Extradural approach to the middle cranial fossa. Positioning and incisions (vertical incision, S-shaped incision)

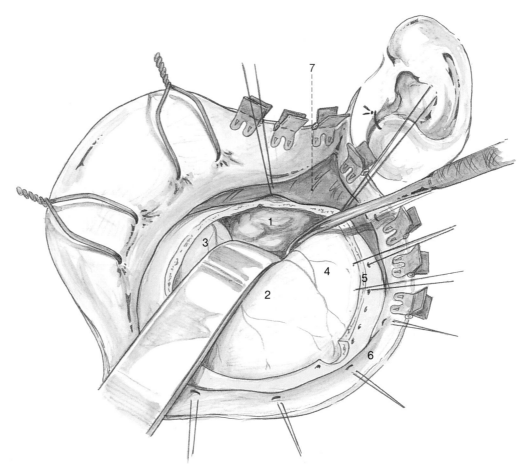

Fig. **80** The bone flap, cut with a craniotome, has been removed. The dura is retracted from the bone with narrow elevators, and is held away with soft spatulas so that the middle cranial fossa is gradually brought into view. The vertical incision has been used. Sutures retract the ear inferiorly

1 Periosteum of the middle cranial fossa, with digitate impressions
2 Dura mater over the temporal lobe
3 Frontal branch of the middle meningeal artery
4 Parietal branch of the middle meningeal artery
5 Circular dural elevation sutures (passed through the bone)
6 Galeal elevation sutures
7 Detached temporal muscle, laterally retracted

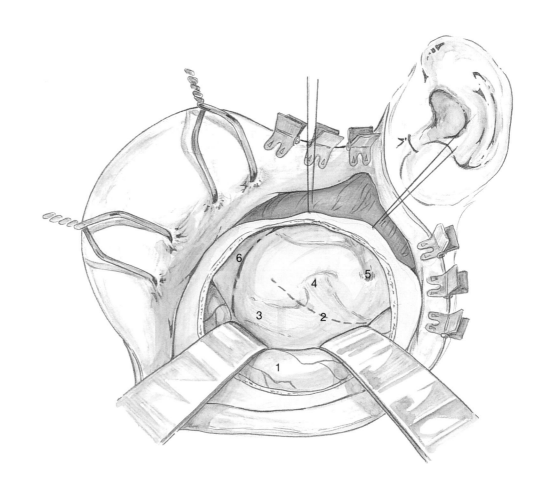

Fig. **81** The trigeminal cavity (Meckel's cavity) can be opened along the broken red line. The structures of the base of the skull are usually hardly visible under the periosteum

1 Dura mater over the temporal lobe
2 Periosteum on the middle cranial fossa, with the incision line
3 Maxillary nerve (foramen rotundum)
4 Mandibular nerve (oval foramen)
5 Middle meningeal artery (spinous foramen)
6 Small sphenoid wing (ala minor ossis sphenoidalis)

Wound Closure

To begin with, the dura is searched for lesions. If such lesions can be exposed, they should be carefully closed by suture. Hereafter, the bone flap is reinserted and approximated with central dural elevation sutures passed through the bone flap. These sutures, together with tight dural elevation sutures at the bone margin, provide the most effective protection against postoperative epidural hematomas.

If necessary, the bone flap can be additionally fixed with nonabsorbable sutures in bone channels at the bone margin. The portions of the temporal muscle are sutured under moderate traction. The fascia of the temporal muscle is approximated. Subcutaneous fatty tissue and skin can be closed with interrupted sutures over a suction drain.

Potential Errors and Dangers

- Overlooked blood loss during the operation due to inadequate hemostasis of the skin flap and its cut border
- Injury of dura and cerebral cortex due to craniotomy instruments
- Injury to a sinus
- Injury to the trigeminal nerve
- Injury to the internal carotid artery in the trigeminal region when there is only a thin lamella or none at all
- Postoperative hemorrhages from inadequately secured dural vessels
- Postoperative epidural hematoma due to inadequate or slack dural elevation sutures
- Soft-tissue hematoma

5 Supratentorial Approaches to the Occipital Region

Occipital-Paramedian Approach to the Occipital Region

Typical Indications for Surgery

– Median tentorial meningiomas
– Tumors of the falcial-tentorial angle
– Arteriovenous malformations
– Inflammatory processes

Principal Anatomical Structures

External occipital protuberance, occipital artery and vein, greater occipital nerve, azygos vein of the neck, galea aponeurotica, occipitofrontal muscle (venter occipitalis), lambdoid suture, dura mater, sagittal sinus, transverse sinus, sinus rectus, confluence of sinuses, arachnoidal granulations, posterior cerebral artery (anterior and posterior branches).

Positioning and Skin Incisions

(Figs. **82, 83**)

The patient's position may be either sitting or prone. Shown here is the procedure in the sitting position. The head should be firmly fixed. It is turned slightly to the side of the lesion so that a better view of the operative field can be obtained. The deeper the process, the smaller the turn required.

The skin incision may be slightly paramedian and serpiginous. The extent of the targeted process may also necessitate an arcuate skin incision going beyond the midline. This permits expansion of the craniotomy to the contralateral side. A precisely marked midline and the external occipital protuberance serve as guides for the skin incision.

After the skin incision, the exposed musculature is incised electrically so that the soft tissues can be broadly retracted from the craniotomy area. The lambdoid suture serves as another landmark.

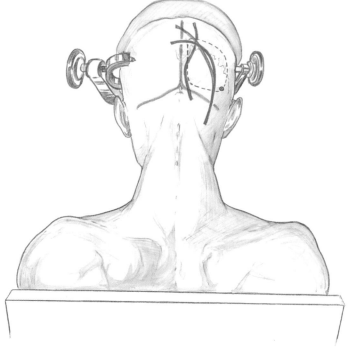

Fig. **82** Occipital-paramedian approach to the occipital region: sitting position and incisions. The border of the bone flap is marked by a black dashed line; the superior sagittal and transverse sinuses are shown in blue. The head is firmly fixed

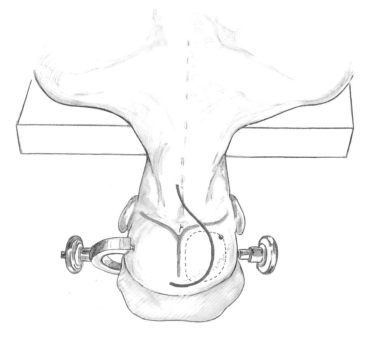

Fig. **83** Occipital-paramedian approach to the occipital region: prone positioning and incision (red). *Black dashed line:* the border of the bone flap; *blue:* the superior sagittal and transverse sinuses. The head is firmly fixed

Craniotomy

(Fig. 84)

One or more burr holes are placed above the transverse sinus; the dura mater is retracted with a Braatz probe or a dissector, and the bone flap is prepared with a craniotome or saw. The borders of the bone flap near the sinus should be sawed open; if there is bleeding from a sinus, the less dangerous bone incisions should already have been made to permit more rapid removal of the bone flap and thus more rapid control of the sinus hemorrhage. The lambdoid suture is crossed in every case. The bone margins close to the sinus are treated with bone wax if necessary in order to avert small air embolisms.

Opening the Dura

The dura is based either in a stellate form in the direction of the transverse and sagittal sinuses, or on one sinus, and is divided at a distance of at least one centimeter from the other sinus. At this point, the exact anatomical location of the craniotomy proves itself; if it is not exact, neither the intercerebral fissure nor the tentorium can be visualized. Dissections performed under such unclear conditions are extremely dangerous. An appropriate osteoclastic expansion of the craniotomy opening then becomes necessary.

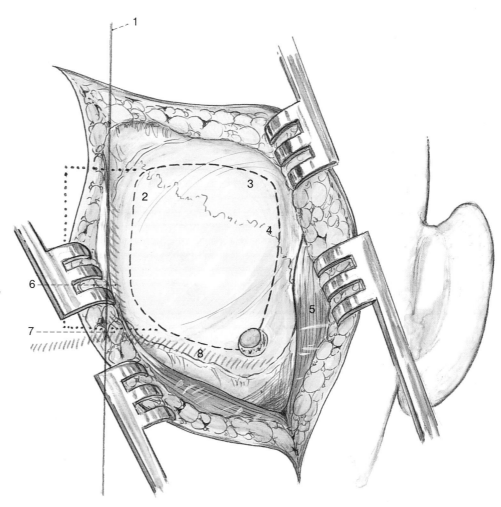

Fig. **84**   The occipital squama has been exposed for craniotomy (dashed line); shown here is the sitting position. *Dotted line:* a possible expansion of the craniotomy beyond the superior sagittal sinus, if this needs to be exposed. The occipitofrontal muscle (venter occipitalis) has been incised longitudinally, and the periosteum has been retracted toward the borders. The midline is clearly marked

1 Midline
2 Occipital bone (superior squama)
3 Parietal bone
4 Lambdoid suture
5 Occipitofrontal muscle (venter occipitalis)
6 Superior sagittal sinus
7 Confluence of the sinuses
8 Transverse sinus

Exposure of the Intercerebral Fissure

(Fig. 85)

Elevation of the brain from the falx and the tentorium has to be carried out with utmost care, because overlooked and subsequently avulsed bridging veins in this area will create problems in hemostasis. If there is no certainty that these veins can be spared, they require bipolar coagulation and division close to the brain and distant from the sinus and

the dura. If coagulation is performed too close to the sinus, holes may be burned into the sinus, resulting in increased bleeding. The desired portion of the occipital lobe is then retracted slowly, step by step, by gentle spatula pressure on the cottonoid-covered brain.

The anatomical relations of the large sinuses in the operative field are depicted in Figure **86**.

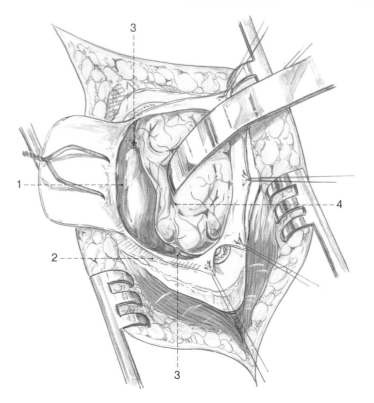

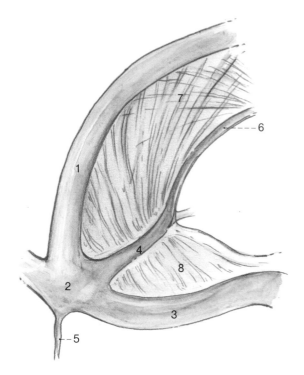

Fig. **85** The dural flap is based in the direction of the longitudinal sinus and reflected. The two adjacent sinuses may just barely be included in the field of vision. The brain has been retracted from the falx; individual bridging veins appear taut

1 Superior sagittal sinus
2 Transverse sinus
3 Bridging veins
4 Calcarine sulcus

Fig. **86** The sinus-falx-tentorium region, right-sided posterolateral view

1 Superior sagittal sinus
2 Confluence of sinuses
3 Transverse sinus
4 Sinus rectus
5 Occipital sagittal sinus
6 Inferior sagittal sinus
7 Falx of the cerebrum
8 Tentorium of the cerebellum

Wound Closure

Following meticulous hemostasis, the necessary dural elevation sutures can be applied. Since the sinus boundaries are difficult to discern, particularly in the sitting position, these elevation sutures are reduced to the absolutely necessary minimum near the superior sagittal sinus and the transverse sinus in order to avoid injury to the sinuses or the sinus lacunae, which may lead to air embolism or rebleeding. The dura itself is closed with interrupted sutures; centrally, the elevation suture is passed through channels in the bone flap. The reimplanted bone flap may receive additional holding sutures of nonabsorbable material. In operations in the sinus region, suction drains, if required at all, should have only weak suction. The divided musculature, the subcutaneous adipose tissue, and the skin are approximated and sutured.

Potential Errors and Dangers

— Overlooked blood loss during the operation due to inadequate hemostasis of the skin flap or its cut border
— Injury to the dura, sinus, or cerebral cortex by craniotomy instruments
— Pressure lesions of the brain due to improper or hasty application of brain spatulas
— Avulsion of noncoagulated bridging veins
— Inadequate closure of veins near sinuses and lacunae
— Postoperative hemorrhages from inadequately secured vessels at the surface of the brain
— Postoperative epidural hematomas due to inadequate or slack dural elevation sutures
— Soft-tissue hematomas

Occipital-Supratentorial Approach to the Occipital Region

Typical Indications for Surgery

- Tumors of the tentorial surface
- Tumors growing supratentorially and infratentorially
- Angiomas
- Meningiomas of the pineal region (see also page 98)
- Inflammatory processes

Principal Anatomical Structures

External occipital protuberance, occipital artery and vein, greater occipital nerve, galea aponeurotica, occipitofrontal muscle (venter occipitalis), temporoparietal muscle, lambdoid suture, dura mater, transverse and superior sagittal sinus, middle cerebral artery (parietal, supramarginal and angular branches), supratentorial bridging veins.

With infratentorial enlargement of the skin incision: Semispinalis capitis, splenius capitis and cervicis muscles; sternocleidomastoid, trapezius and posterior auricular muscles; dorsal branches of cervical nerves 3–5 (cutaneous branches); dura mater; transverse, rectus, and occipital sinuses; infratentorial bridging veins, pineal region, deep cerebral veins (internal and great cerebral veins, basal and posterior cerebral veins).

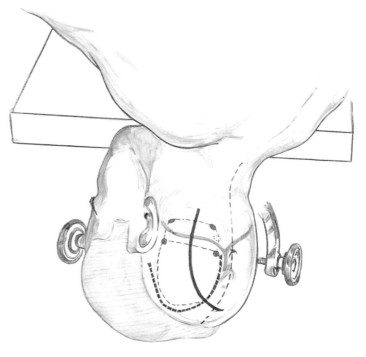

Fig. **87** Occipital-supratentorial approach to the supratentorial occipital region: positioning and incision. *Black dashed line:* the border of the bone flap; caudally adjoining is a possible expansion toward the cerebellar area. *Blue:* the adjacent sinuses

Positioning and Skin Incisions
(Fig. **87**)

The patient is placed in prone position, or on his or her side, and the head is firmly fixed, slightly turned, and tilted downward. Thus, the middle of the craniotomy site is at the highest point.

The skin incision may be made either supratentorially, describing an arc with the stalk heading toward the transverse sinus, or it may be crescent-shaped, passing from the lateral nuchal area across the midline to the contralateral occipital region.

The choice depends on the extent to which the craniotomy may be expanded into the infratentorial region. The procedure described below includes this infratentorial expansion; accordingly, the semicircular incision is shown.

An attempt is made to spare the greater occipital nerve and accompanying vessels; in the majority of operations this cannot be done. Using cutting diathermy, the muscle is dissected from the bone and drawn out of the operative field with retractors. The external occipital protuberance and the lambdoid suture serve as anatomical landmarks.

Craniotomy
(Fig. 88)

Burr holes are placed just above the transverse sinus and at a point nearly 2 cm from the superior sagittal sinus. A craniotome or saw is used to cut oblique edges around the bone flap, starting at the borders remote from the sinus. If the craniotomy has to be expanded in the infratentorial direction, infratentorial burr holes are placed near and parallel to the transverse sinus, and the craniotome then cuts around the adjoining bone flap. Not infrequently, the danger of injury to the dura and sinus makes it necessary to perform the enlargement toward the posterior cranial fossa osteoclastically. Oozing hemorrhages from the undamaged transverse sinus are controlled by application of hemostatic materials and tamponades. Injuries to the sinus require sealing with dura or muscle fragments and added use of fibrin adhesive.

Opening the Dura
(Fig. 89)

The supratentorial dural flap is based toward the superior sagittal sinus. In the direction of the transverse sinus, there remains a strip of dura at least one centimeter wide that is joined to an equally wide infratentorial strip with several interrupted sutures over the transverse sinus to protect the sinus in the further course of the operation. Thus, the infratentorial dural incision is U-shaped, with the stalk directed toward the sinus.

In the next step, the occipital pole is cautiously lifted off the tentorium, and is detached from the falx at the same time. The highly variable bridging veins have to be brought into view; whether they can be spared needs to be determined in each individual case. If they have to be divided, use is made of duplicate bipolar coagulation, again close to the brain and far from the dura. Possible courses of veins at and in the tentorium are suggested in Figure **90**.

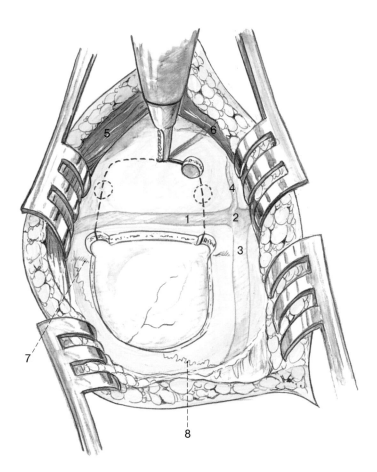

Fig. **88** The supratentorial craniotomy has been completed, and the caudally adjoining bone over the cerebellum is circumferentially incised with a craniotome after retraction of the transverse sinus with Braatz probes

1 Transverse sinus
2 Confluence of the sinuses
3 Superior sagittal sinus
4 Occipital sinus
5 Trapezius muscle
6 Semispinalis capitis muscle
7 Superior nuchal line
8 Lambdoid suture

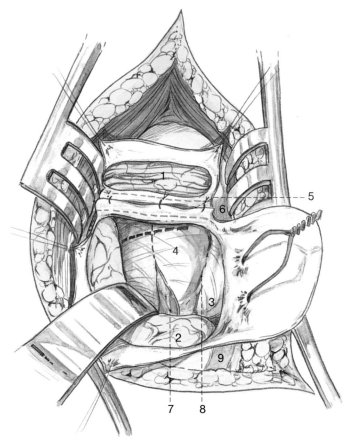

Fig. **89** The supratentorial dural flap is based in the direction of the longitudinal sinus and reflected; the infratentorial dural flap is based caudally and elevated by suture. The dural segments adjacent to the transverse sinus are temporarily sutured over the sinus for its protection. After this, the medial portion of the occipital flap can be retracted laterally-superiorly, so that the tentorium is brought into view. A longitudinal and transverse incision into it causes the adjacent infratentorial structures to be visualized

1 Cerebellum
2 Calcarine sulcus
3 Falx of cerebrum
4 Tentorium of cerebellum (partly incised)
5 Transverse sinus (protected by dura)
6 Confluence of the sinuses
7 Great cerebral vein (Galen's vein) and internal cerebral veins
8 Sinus rectus
9 Superior sagittal sinus

If incision of the tentorium becomes necessary, an incision toward the tentorial notch is connected with a transverse incision made close to the transverse sinus.

When infratentorial trephination has been performed at the same time, a combined supratentorial and infratentorial procedure is now possible.

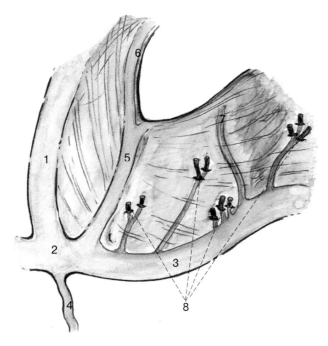

Fig. **90**   Veins between the tentorium and the cerebral surface, right-sided posterolateral view

1 Superior sagittal sinus
2 Confluence of sinuses
3 Transverse sinus
4 Occipital sinus
5 Sinus rectus
6 Inferior sagittal sinus
7 Superior petrosal sinus
8 Inferior cerebral veins (marked variations occur)

Wound Closure

Owing to the usual relief of pressure, the dura can usually be closed with interrupted sutures without difficulty. If an appropriate, tight dural closure – particularly over the cerebellum in the expanded procedure – is not possible, dural reconstruction with autologous fascia lata or lyophilized dura is advisable. In the presence of inflammatory processes, exogenous materials ought not to be employed. Unless the brain pressure precludes it, the bone flap is reinserted, fixed with nonabsorbable retention sutures, and the central dural elevation suture on the bone flap is tied with requisite caution. Suction drains with low suction should be used in operations close to the sinus only if absolutely necessary. The subcutis is approximated with absorbable material, and the skin is closed with sutures or metal clamps.

Potential Errors and Dangers

— Overlooked blood loss during the operation due to inadequate hemostasis of the skin flap and its cut borders
— Injury to the dura and cerebral cortex due to craniotomy instruments
— Cerebral pressure lesions due to improper and hasty application of brain spatulas
— Injury to a sinus or its lacunae
— Avulsion of bridging veins
— Postoperative hemorrhages from unsecured vessels at the brain surface
— Postoperative epidural hematoma due to inadequate or slack dural elevation sutures
— Soft-tissue hematoma

6 Direct Approach to the Occipital Region

Occipital Transcerebral Approach to the Occipital Region

Typical Indications for Surgery

- Tumors in the occipital cerebral lobe
- Angiomas in the occipital region
- Processes in the posterior horn of the lateral ventricle

Principal Anatomical Structures

Azygos vein of neck, occipital artery and vein, greater and lesser occipital nerve, epicranial muscle (venter occipitalis), sternocleidomastoid muscle, trapezius muscle, tendinous arch, semispinalis capitis muscle, splenius capitis muscle, external occipital protuberance, nuchal line, occipital bone (superior and inferior squama), lambdoid suture, sagittal suture, occipital diploic vein, dura mater, transverse sinus, superior sagittal sinus, sinus rectus, occipital veins, parieto-occipital and calcarine branches of the middle occipital artery, occipital gyri, parieto-occipital sulcus, lunate sulcus, calcarine sulcus, occipital and preoccipital striate areas.

Positioning and Skin Incision

(Fig. 91)

The patient may be placed in a prone position, on the side, in sitting position or, as described below, in a supine position. Each position has its advantages and disadvantages. Additionally, anesthetic requirements need to be considered in the individual patient. Finally, body weight, muscle mass, and the mobility of the cervical spine enter into the choice of position. Therefore, it is inadvisable to become accustomed to one particular type of positioning, even if a certain position is usually given preference. In all cases, the positioning must permit the use of optical enlargement,

optimal illumination, and other essential techniques of microneurosurgery. Firm fixation of the head is frequently helpful.

The skin incision over the occipital region has the typical arcuate shape, and is based laterally or, as described below, medially. With medial stalking, the incision tends to cross the midline.

Craniotomy

(Fig. 92)

With the chosen type of incision, the nuchal muscles are not included in the operative field, but remain immediately adjacent to it. In the majority of cases, the occipital artery cannot be spared; however, the greater occipital nerve should be prepared and displaced laterally. The lambdoid suture runs obliquely through the exposed cranial region. Behind it, a single burr hole is placed if a craniotome is used to prepare the bone flap. With the use of the Gigli saw, a number of burr holes are required. Injury to the superior longitudinal sinus is avoided by keeping a distance of about one centimeter from the midline. Use of the Braatz probe to retract the dura from the bone is important, especially in the area of the lambdoid suture. The bone flap is freed from the subjacent dural surface with an elevator, and is packed off under moist and warm conditions during the operation.

Opening the Dura and Incision of the Brain

(Fig. 93)

The base of the excised dural flap is similarly directed toward the sagittal sinus. The incision is made at a distance of several millimeters from the bone margin to facilitate final suture of the dura. Tangential incisions and corresponding elevation sutures allow full utilization of the craniotomy.

The approach to the brain generally makes use of the nearest sulcus, unless special functions of this region forbid it (Fig. 94).

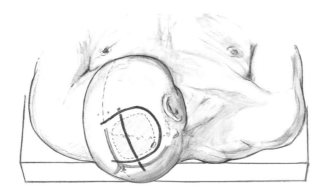

Fig. **91** Approach to the occipital region: positioning and incision. The skin incision may also have a lateral base. *Black dashes:* the border of the bone flap; the top is shaded. *Blue:* the superior sagittal sinus and the transverse sinus. Only the external occipital protuberance is palpable

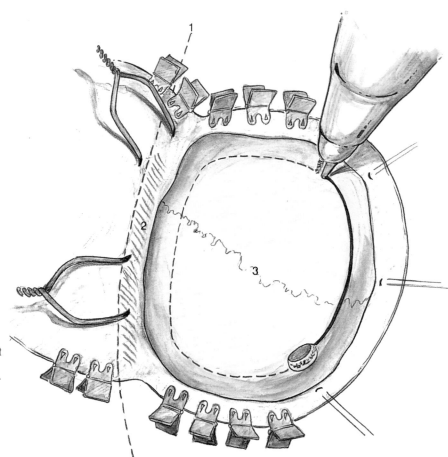

Fig. **92** The skin flap is opened medially: the galea is retracted laterally by strong sutures. After placement of one or more burr holes, a cut is made around the bone flap. The lambdoid suture provides a bony landmark. The midline is clearly marked on the skin to avoid injury to the superior sagittal sinus

1 Midline
2 Superior sagittal sinus
3 Lambdoid suture

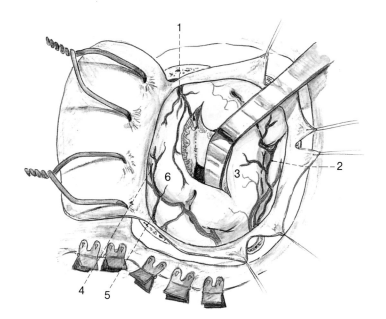

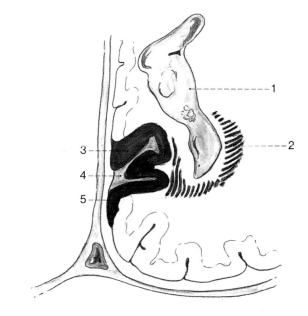

Fig. **93** After being incised, the dura is reflected toward the middle, and elevation sutures are placed in its corners. The cerebral cortex is entered in the region of the selected sulcus, and the tumor is becoming barely visible. The brain spatulas are applied gently and elastically

1 Precuneal artery
2 Posterior temporal artery
3 Inferior parietal lobule
4 Parieto-occipital sulcus
5 Parieto-occipital branch of the posterior cerebral artery
6 Superior parietal lobule

Fig. **94** The anatomical relations between the visual cortex (brown) and the lateral ventricle

1 Posterior horn of the lateral ventricle
2 Optic radiation
3 Striate cortex (upper lip)
4 Calcarine sulcus
5 Striate cortex (lower lip)

Wound Closure

Suture of the dura, using interrupted sutures in most cases, can be carried out only after meticulous hemostasis in all the exposed segments (this may include the medial surface of the occipital lobe). Continuous suture may be used as well but this requires intermittent tying every 2–3 cm. Next to be placed are the dural elevation sutures to prevent postoperative epidural hematoma; it is safest to pass these sutures through separate bone channels.

The bone flap to be reimplanted also receives central burr holes, through which additional dural elevation sutures are drawn; they are designed for prevention of hematomas as well as for fixation of the bone flap. This fixation may be reinforced by retention sutures that are passed longitudinally from both galeal-periosteal areas. The need for insertion of a suction drain has to be decided from case to case.

The operation is completed by placement of interrupted sutures for the skin.

Potential Errors and Dangers

— Overlooked blood loss due to inadequate hemostasis in the area of the skin flap
— Avoidable injury to the greater occipital nerve
— Dural injury due to craniotomy instruments
— Brain damage due to overly vigorous application of brain spatulas
— Avoidable injury to functionally important brain regions
— Postoperative epidural hematoma due to inadequate or slack dural elevation sutures
— Soft-tissue hematoma due to inadequate cutaneous hemostasis

7 Approaches to the Anterior Midline Region

Transfrontal Transventricular Approach to the Anterior Midline Region

Typical Indications for Surgery

— Tumors of the anterior portions of the lateral ventricle
— Tumors in the deep anterior cerebral medulla
— Tumors and cysts in the anterior portions of the third ventricle

Principal Anatomical Structures

Galea aponeurotica, superficial temporal artery (frontal branch), supraorbital nerve (lateral branch), frontal bone (squama), frontal sinus, middle meningeal artery (frontal branch), frontal diploic vein, dura mater, superior middle and inferior frontal gyrus, lateral frontobasal artery (from the middle cerebral artery), frontal horn of the lateral ventricle, interventricular foramen, head of the caudate nucleus, pellucid septum, choroid plexus of the lateral ventricle, posterior vein of the pellucid septum, superior thalamostriate vein, anterior vein of the pellucid septum, arteria pericallosa.

Positioning and Skin Incisions
(Fig. 95)

The patient is placed in a supine position, and the head is turned to the contralateral side by about 30 degrees. It is fixed in a headrest, with the single pin lying on the side of the operation, for procedures involving use of the microscope.

The skin incision is usually semiarcuate, running from within the hairline 2–3 cm lateral to the midline to a point slightly above the anterior border of the ear; it therefore runs parallel to a portion of the coronal suture and ends at the sphenofrontal suture. Cosmetic considerations may dictate a preference for the Unterberger incision.

Dissection of Soft Tissues

The skin flap is dissected free using blunt dissection – with a flat scalpel blade only for the basal portions – until the desired craniotomy area has been exposed. A fishhook or an elevation suture keeps it safely outside the operative field. In the next step, the galea aponeurotica is incised, and this once again is done very delicately, in case this layer should be needed for reconstructive purposes at the end of the operation. The fishhooks or elevation sutures are transferred to this galeal flap. Three to four retention sutures, which enlarge the approach and facilitate the craniotomy per se, are placed in the narrow galeal portions at the remaining cut border.

Craniotomy
(Fig. 96)

Here, the customary four or five drill holes, subsequently joined by means of the Gigli saw, may be used unless a single burr hole and subsequent use of the craniotome are preferred. The shape of the bone flap to be turned is also determined by the size of the frontal sinus, and its size by the location of the target object and the surgeon's experience. During the operation, the bone flap is packed away under sterile, moist conditions.

Opening the Dura
(Fig. 97)

The incision of the dura, directed toward the midline, is made about one centimeter inward from the craniotomy bone margin. Tangential incisions are used to take full advantage of the bone opening; the dural flaps are lifted up with fine sutures. At this site, too, dural elevation sutures passing through the bone should be placed, but not tied, before or immediately after incision of the dura. .

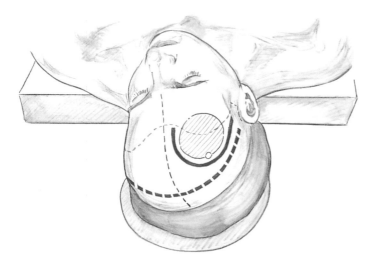

Fig. **95** Transfrontal transventricular approach to the structures of the anterior midline: positioning and incisions (arcuate incision, U-shaped incision). *Black:* the border of the bone flap. *Shading:* the bone flap itself. *Black dashed line:* usual hairline. The arcuate incision is presented in the figures below

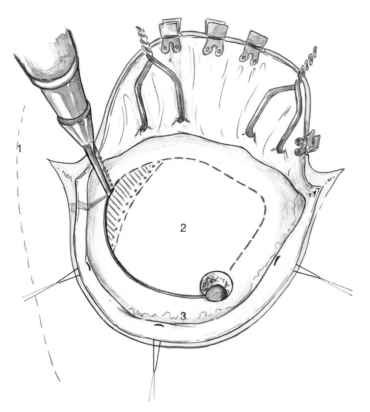

Fig. **96** Starting from one burr hole, a craniotome cut is made around the bone flap. In the presence of very extensive frontal sinuses, a smaller craniotomy may become necessary, meaning that the red-shaded area is left in place. The coronal suture aids further orientation on the bone

1 Midline
2 Craniotomy of reduced size (dotted line: burr line)
3 Coronal suture

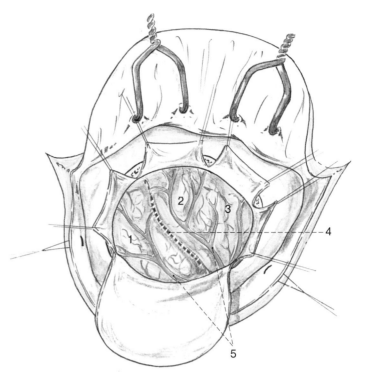

Fig. **97** The dura has been incised and reflected dorsally; its corners are elevated by sutures. The brain can now be entered in the preselected sulcus (dotted red line)

1 Superior frontal gyrus   4 Superior frontal sulcus
2 Middle frontal gyrus   5 Frontal veins
3 Inferior frontal gyrus

Dissection of the Brain and Opening of the Lateral Ventricle

(Fig. 98)

To begin with, the arachnoid is opened under the surgical microscope, usually in the anterior frontal sulcus. After retraction of the vessels, dissection may proceed bluntly and with a few bipolar coagulations in the direction of the anterior horn of the lateral ventricle. A safeguard is provided by prior measurement of the computed tomogram; alternatively, intradural sonography may be employed.

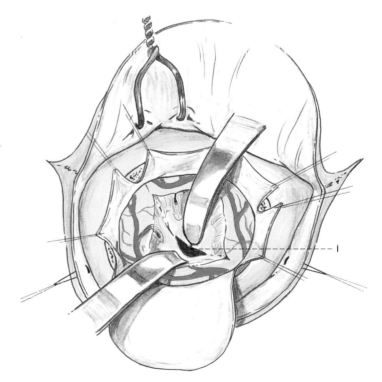

Fig. **98** The brain is retracted with narrow, soft spatulas until the anterior horn of the right lateral ventricle is reached

1 Anterior horn of the lateral ventricle

Exploration of the Interventricular Foramen and Third Ventricle

(Fig. 99)

With optimal illumination and narrow binocular inspection, the anatomical structures in the ventricles are as readily identifiable as cysts and tumors. As a rule, the interventricular foramen is widened or even considerably dilated by masses in the third ventricle, while the wall of the cyst or tumor protrudes directly through the foramen into the lateral ventricle. The preconditions for operating on these masses are therefore met.

In the case of deep-seated tumors of the cerebral medulla, the surgeon passes the contralateral ventricular wall and exposes the tumor. Intraoperative sonography is extremely helpful in this situation.

The anatomical conditions inside the lateral ventricles are readily discernible. The veins entering the internal cerebral vein are clearly visualized, as are the most anterior parts of the choroid plexus (Fig. 100). Local deformities of whole ventricles or parts of them can result both from direct tumor pressure and from a preexisting obstructive hydrocephalus.

Final closure of the ventricular wall rarely succeeds, but is hardly ever necessary. If the superficial arachnoid can be sealed, this will prevent postoperative effusions, which are not uncommon.

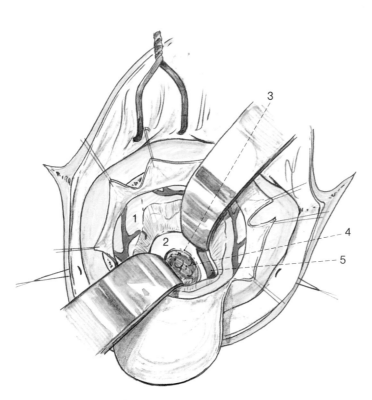

Fig. **99** When the lateral ventricle has been exposed with the aid of self-retaining soft spatulas, the interventricular foramen and the tumor are brought into view

1 Superior frontal gyrus
2 Anterior horn of the right lateral ventricle
3 Dilated interventricular foramen
4 Wall of a colloid cyst
5 Septal vein

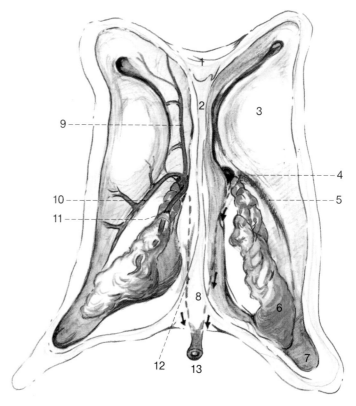

Fig. **100** Anatomy of the veins in the area of the interventricular foramen. Viewed from above, the confluence of the septum pellucidum veins, superior thalamostriate veins, and the middle superior choroid veins to form the left and right internal cerebral vein is clearly visualized. In the area of pulvinar thalami, an additional vein (the middle thalamostriate vein) may in some cases run through the lamina affixa toward the internal cerebral vein, or may open directly into the great cerebral vein

1 Genu of the corpus callosum
2 Pellucid septum
3 Head of the caudate nucleus
4 Interventricular foramen
5 Thalamus and lamina affixa
6 Choroid plexus
7 Occipital horn of the lateral ventricle and the collateral trigone
8 Splenium corporis callosi
9 Posterior vein of the pellucid septum
10 Superior thalamostriate vein
11 Middle superior choroid vein
12 Internal cerebral vein
13 Great cerebral vein

Bone and Wound Closure

Following the customary dural suture and tying of the dural elevation sutures, the bone flap is fixed in its craniotomy opening by means of central dural elevation sutures passed through the bone, or by tension sutures, or both. The reflected galea may be used for free or pedicled reconstruction of the dura as well as for covering osteoclastic defects. No additional sutures are otherwise needed.

After a final and careful inspection and, if necessary, introduction of a subcutaneous suction drain, the skin is closed with interrupted sutures.

Potential Errors and Dangers

— Overlooked blood loss due to inadequate hemostasis in the cutaneous region
— Dural injuries due to the craniotomy instruments
— Pressure lesions of the brain due to excessively harsh use of brain spatulas
— Additional parenchymal lesions due to a repeated approach to very small lateral ventricles (sonography)
— Injuries of contiguous midline structures
— Postoperative epidural hematoma due to inadequate or slack dural elevation sutures
— Soft-tissue hematoma

Transcallosal Approach to the Anterior Midline Region

Typical Indications for Surgery

— Neoplasms in the anterior part of the third ventricle (astrocytomas, colloid cysts, ependymal cysts, craniopharyngiomas, etc.)
— Deep-seated vascular malformations

Principal Anatomical Structures

Galea aponeurotica, superficial temporal artery (frontal branch), supraorbital nerve (lateral branch), frontal bone (squama), frontal sinus, middle meningeal artery (frontal branch), frontal diploic vein, dura mater, superior sagittal sinus, inferior sagittal sinus, cerebral falx, superior frontal gyrus, gyrus cinguli, corpus callosum, arteria pericallosa, callosomarginal artery, anterior cerebral veins, terminal lamina, body of the fornix, third ventricle, adhesio interthalamica.

Positioning and Skin Incisions
(Fig. 101)

The patient is in a supine position with the head firmly restrained. During the operation, the head may have to be

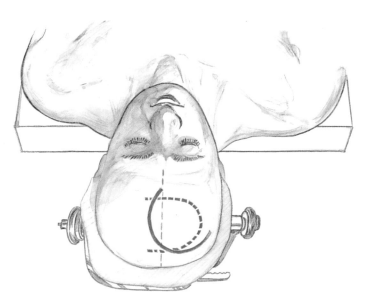

Fig. **101** Transcallosal approach to structures of the anterior midline: positioning and incisions (arcuate incision with laterobasal pedicle, arcuate incision with medial pedicle). Both incisions cross the midline. The head is firmly fixed. In the following figures, use is made of the laterobasally pedicled incision.

turned 10–15 degrees toward the contralateral side; for this purpose, the operating table is tilted sideways, unless use is made of a highly mobile surgical microscope.

One possible skin incision is arcuate, curving across the midline and heading in a laterobasal direction (solid line in Fig. **101**). An alternative is an incision from the contralateral side, with the flap being based toward the contralateral side (dashed line in Fig. **101**). If there are cosmetic problems, a bow-shaped incision from the beginning of one ear to the other may be made, the skin flap being retracted toward the orbit.

In every case, even small hemorrhages should be carefully controlled at the beginning of the operation, without relying on the uncertain effect of clamps or clips. Otherwise, sizable amounts of blood could ooze out during the ensuing operation without attracting notice. This warning should be taken particularly seriously in children.

Dissection of Soft Tissues

The skin flap is retracted in the layer between the galea and the periosteum in familiar fashion, using a flat scalpel blade or pledgets, so that tissue will remain available for a possible reconstruction. After the incision, the periosteum, too, is retracted toward the base of the flap. The layers are kept out of the operative field with fishhooks or elevation sutures. Three to five retention sutures, which enlarge the purposely restricted approach, are placed in the narrow galeal areas at the border (Fig. **102**).

Craniotomy
(Fig. **102**)

Generally speaking, a single, laterally placed burr hole followed by craniotome preparation of the bone flap may suffice. However, since the craniotomy is generally extended beyond the superior sagittal sinus, so that the risk of a sinus injury by the burr cannot be dismissed, it is advisable to place burr holes on both sides of the sinus at distances of about 1.5 cm from the midline. Through these burr holes, it is nearly always possible to retract the sinus with Braatz probes without injury, so that the craniotome or Gigli saw over the watchspring probe will not collide with the longitudinal sinus. The surgeon's individual experience will be the determining factor in these situations. The bone flap is now carefully detached from the dura with blunt elevators and is packed off under sterile, moist conditions during the ensuing operation. Not uncommonly, there will be bleeding from small venous orifices over and alongside the sinus after removal of the bone flap. Bipolar coagulation may be used to stop the bleeding, but this leads to local contraction of the dura. Application of hemostatic material patches, such as Tabotamp, for example, is preferable. At the end of the operation, these small hemorrhages have usually permanently stopped as a result. The midline, which should be drawn in, is the most important landmark for the operation. The coronal suture is likewise helpful.

Opening the Dura
(Fig. **103**)

The arcuate dura incision which is made at a distance of barely one centimeter from the craniotomy border is directed toward the sinus; it is brought closer to the conduit with very small cuts, since so-called lacunae may bulge out from the sinus, so that hemorrhages are provoked. By extending beyond the sinus, the craniotomy may cause the midline region to be displaced several millimeters toward the contralateral side, the consequence being that the mid-

line approach is considerably improved. Veins between the brain surface and the sinus ought to be spared whenever possible. Whether one or the other vessel may have to be removed depends on the requirements of the subsequent approach.

Exploration of the Corpus Callosum
(Fig. **104**)

Self-retaining spatulas, applied with little pressure, gradually retract the hemisphere outward millimeter by millimeter. The same procedure is followed for the falx. This brings into view the corpus callosum, which is immediately identifiable by its color and vascular pattern. The corpus callosum is incised with a fine knife or a laser beam between the two arteries coursing adjacent to its midline (dashed line in Fig. **104**). The anatomical conditions are illustrated in Figure **105** (cerebral falx and adjacent cerebral sinuses) and Figure **106** (corpus callosum and fornix viewed from the right side).

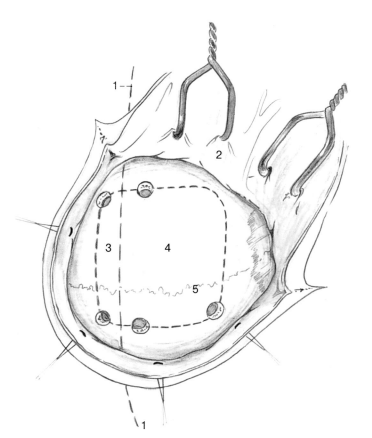

Fig. **102**   The skin flap is reflected and the galea drawn laterally with retention sutures. The osseous fixation point is the coronal suture; the midline is exactly marked on the scalp to permit precise localization of the burr holes next to the superior sagittal sinus

1 Midline
2 Galea aponeurotica
3 Left part of the bone flap
4 Right part of the bone flap
5 Coronal suture

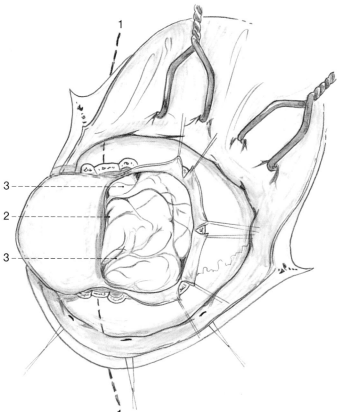

Fig. **103**   An incision has been made around the dura, forming a medial base, nearly reaching the superior sagittal sinus. The individual conditions in the falx-sinus region, and particularly the position and number of bridging veins, can be inspected

1 Midline
2 Superior sagittal sinus
3 Frontal superficial cerebral veins

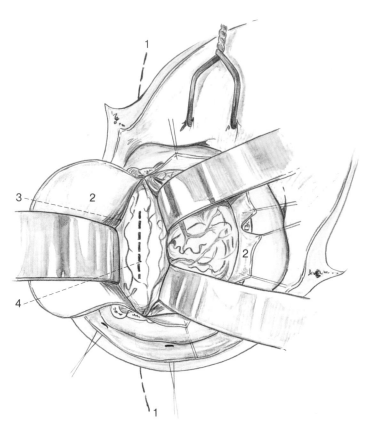

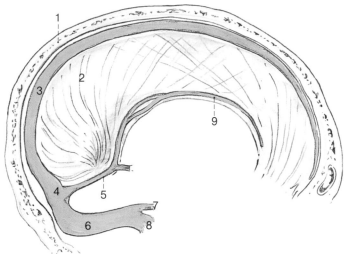

Fig. **104** With the aid of self-retaining spatulas, the falx and superior sagittal sinus are retracted medially, and the brain laterally. As a result, the surface of the corpus callosum is brought into view. *Red dashed line:* the proposed incision site

1 Midline
2 Dura mater
3 Superior sagittal sinus
4 Corpus callosum, with the incision line

Fig. **105** Anatomy of the falx cerebri and adjacent sinuses. In the median and anterior regions of the falx, bridging veins may open into the superior sagittal sinus, as well as into its lateral lacunae

1 Calvaria
2 Falx of cerebrum
3 Superior sagittal sinus
4 Confluence of the sinuses
5 Sinus rectus
6 Transverse sinus
7 Superior petrosal sinus
8 Sigmoid sinus
9 Inferior sagittal sinus

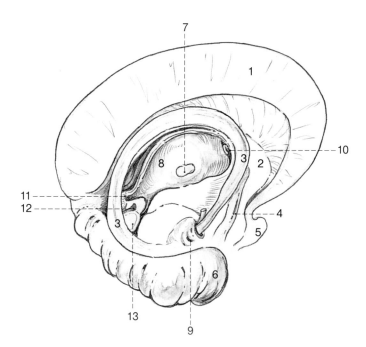

Fig. **106** Corpus callosum and fornix. The lateral wall of the lateral and third ventricles has been removed in order to display the course of the fibers of the right fornix from the mamillary bodies to the fimbria of the fornix, and the hippocampus. The corpus callosum, terminal lamina, optic chiasm, and supraoptic recess have been divided in the midline

1 Corpus callosum
2 Pellucid septum
3 Fornix with columna, crus, and fimbria hippocampi
4 Rostral commissure
5 Optic nerve
6 Hippocampus
7 Adhesio interthalamica
8 Third ventricle
9 Mamillary body
10 Interventricular foramen
11 Pineal body
12 Commissure of the epithalamus
13 Tectum of the mesencephalon

Exploration of the Fornix
(Fig. **107**)

After completion of this incision of the corpus callosum, the fornix bodies are visualized. Once again, the incision is made in a longitudinal direction, so that the third ventricle is brought into view. This completes the approach to a targeted third ventricle tumor.

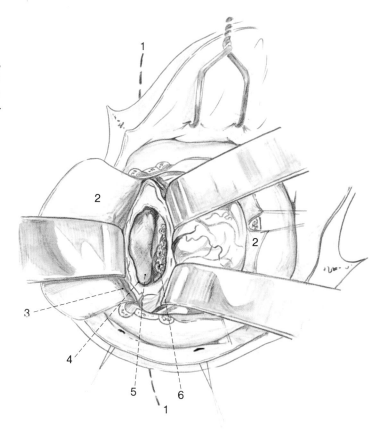

Fig. **107**   The corpus callosum has been incised longitudinally, so that the fornix and the choroid plexus in the third ventricle are visualized

1 Midline
2 Dura mater
3 Superior sagittal sinus
4 Corpus callosum (incised)
5 Fornix
6 Choroid plexus

Bone and Wound Closure

The familiar interrupted-suture closure of the dura, with tying of the dural elevation sutures passing through bone channels that were placed at the start of the craniotomy, is followed by reimplantation of the bone flap. Before this, hemostasis in the sinus region should be verified once again. Fixation of the bone flap can be effected with central dural elevation sutures passed through the bone, or with longitudinal retention sutures, or both.

The skin is usually closed with interrupted sutures.

Potential Errors and Dangers

— Overlooked blood loss due to inadequate cutaneous hemostasis
— Dural injuries during craniotomy
— Injuries to the superior sagittal sinus
— Pressure lesions of the brain due to overly harsh application of brain spatulas
— Excessive division of the corpus callosum
— Postoperative epidural hematoma due to inadequate or slack dural elevation sutures
— Soft-tissue hematomas due to inadequate hemostasis of the skin

Subfrontal Transterminal Approach to the Anterior Midline Region

Typical Indications for Surgery

— Tumors in the basal area of the third ventricle, notably craniopharyngiomas
— Subchiasmal tumors of varying histology
— Retrochiasmal tumors

Principal Anatomical Structures

Galea aponeurotica, superficial temporal artery (frontal branch), supratrochlear vein, supraorbital nerve (lateral branch), frontal bone (squama), frontal sinus, frontal diploic vein, middle meningeal artery (frontal branch), dura mater, superior and inferior sagittal sinus, cerebral falx, superior and middle frontal gyrus, superior cerebral veins, gyrus cinguli, anterior cranial fossa, crista galli, olfactory bulb and tract, optic nerve and chiasm, anterior cerebral artery, anterior communicating artery, sellar tubercle, terminal lamina, pituitary and hypophyseal stalk, diaphragm of the sella turcica.

Positioning and Skin Incisions
(Fig. **108**)

Since a craniotomy crossing the sagittal sinus frequently becomes necessary, a U-shaped incision from the beginning of one ear to the other is recommended. The patient is placed in supine position, with the head slightly flexed. As a rule, the head is rigidly fixed.

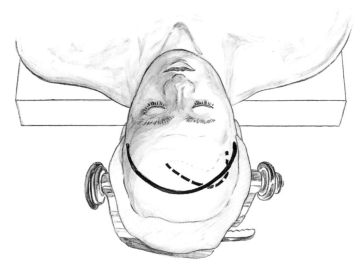

Fig. **108** Subfrontal transterminal approach to the anterior midline: positioning and incisions (overlapping arcuate incision, horseshoe incision). The head is firmly fixed. The illustrations below feature the horseshoe incision

However, the incision may also be in the shape of a hockey stick. It starts beyond the midline at the hairline and extends across the frontal tuber to the anterior temporal region (broken line in Fig. **108**). The head should then be turned about ten degrees to the contralateral side.

Particular attention is paid to the galeal layer, which may be needed for possible reconstruction, and to the control of all hemorrhages, even minor ones. The skin flap is retracted with a fishhook or with elevation sutures, while the other cut borders are secured with retention sutures.

Craniotomy
(Fig. **109**)

If the sagittal sinus is not crossed, placement of one burr hole and subsequent passage of a craniotome around the bone flap will be sufficient. In a procedure going beyond the sinus, additional burr holes should be placed at a distance of about 1.5 cm on both sides of the sinus. This permits the sinus to be retracted from the bone with Braatz probes, so that use of the Gigli saw or a craniotome will not cause any injury to the sagittal sinus or to tributary veins. Removal of the bone flap nearly always necessitates separation of periosteum and dura with an elevator. The bone flap is then packed off in a sterile and moist environment. There usually will be bleeding over the sagittal sinus from a few, generally small, venous openings. Application of hemostatic cloth is preferable to bipolar coagulation, which leads to local shrinkage of the dura.

The midline, which should be drawn in, is the most important landmark.

Opening the Dura
(Fig. **110**)

The basic scheme is a U-shaped dural incision performed one centimeter from the craniotomy border, to which relief incisions are added. Elevation sutures through the corners of the dura provide maximal exposure of the operative field.

Twofold ligation of the superior sagittal sinus in its anterior portion is critical for the bilateral procedure, and makes separation of the falx possible. The procedure is shown in the inset figure at the lower right: under good illumination, the dural incision that is carried as far as the sinus is developed into the cerebral falx below the conduit; a suitable round needle is run through the falx, and the heavy suture is tied over the dura. This step is repeated more centrally at a distance of 1.5 cm. This completes the dural incision, including division of the sinus, and permits division of the adjoining falx. In this area, the inferior sagittal sinus can usually be controlled by bipolar coagulation.

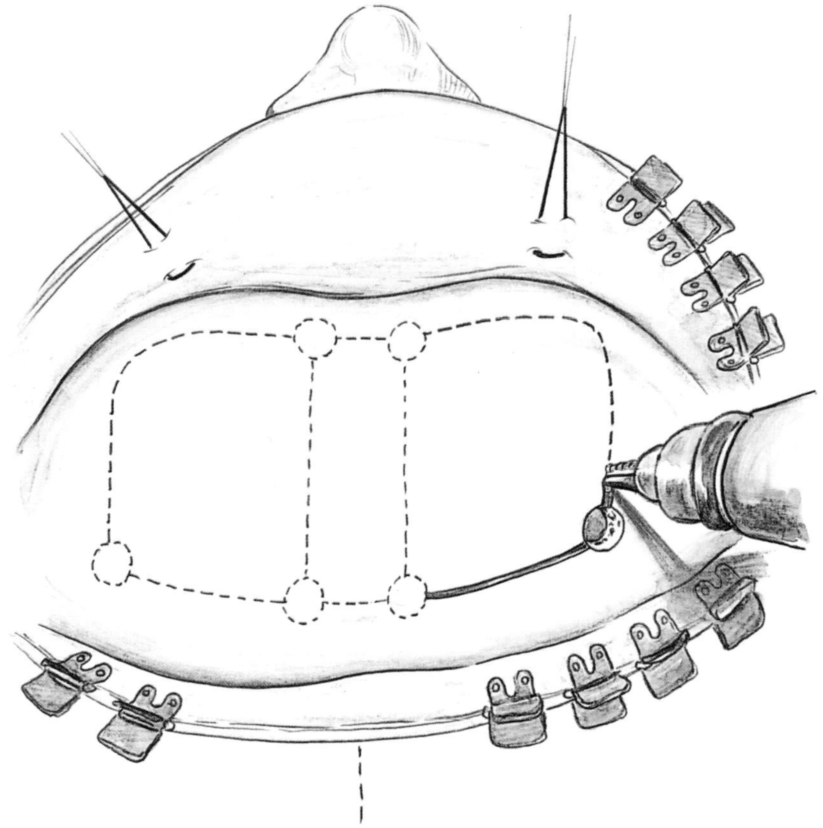

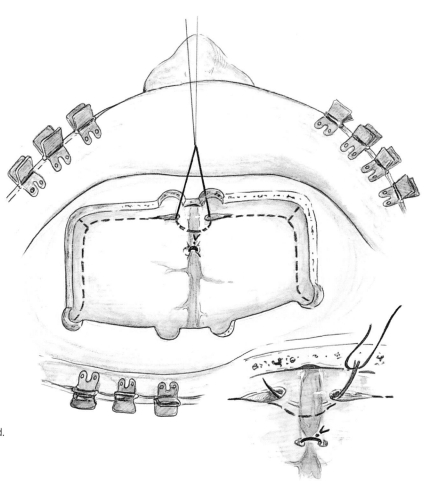

Fig. **109** Both the unilateral and the bilateral procedure are shown. In the vicinity of the superior sagittal sinus, it is always advisable to place additional burr holes, so that the dura-invested sinus can be retracted from the inner surface of the bone

Fig. **110** The solid bone flap has been removed. Incision of the dura begins on both sides of the superior sagittal sinus and anteriorly, so that the sinus can be doubly ligated. After this, the sinus and the adjoining falx can be divided. The inset shows a piercing ligature of the sinus and a second knotted suture. *Red dashed line:* the dural incision

After completed division of the falx (Fig. 111) the dural flap can be reflected, underpadded, and covered. It may be left in place to serve as a natural brain covering. In the further course of the procedure, it is now possible to elevate one or both frontal lobe poles and also to distract them.

Incision of the Terminal Lamina
(Fig. 112)

Exposure of the retrochiasmal area requires optimal relief of tension in the surrounding brain by dehydration and drainage of cerebrospinal fluid. Besides the optic structures, the local vessels in particular enter the field of vision. The terminal lamina lying directly behind the chiasm may be extended anteriorly by a tumor situated behind it; it then tends to be markedly thicker than it normally is. The incision of the lamina is carried out with a fine scalpel, bipolar coagulation and cooling, microforceps, or by laser. The importance of substantial magnification with the surgical microscope cannot be overemphasized.

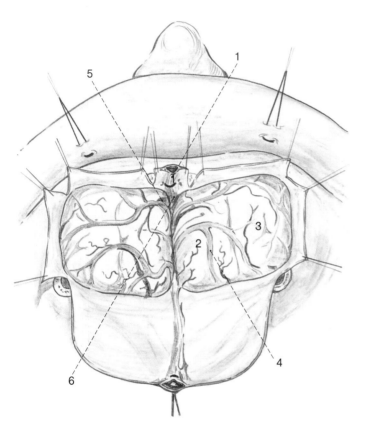

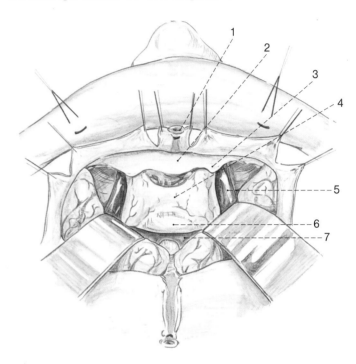

Fig. 111   The dural flap has been reflected posteriorly, but it can also be left in place to serve as a natural protection for the brain. The two frontal lobe poles can now be elevated

1 Superior sagittal sinus (transected)
2 Superior frontal gyrus
3 Middle frontal gyrus
4 Frontal superior cerebral veins
5 Medial frontal branches of callosomarginal artery
6 Cerebral falx (divided)

Fig. 112   The two frontal lobe poles have been elevated and retracted. This gives access to a view into the anterior cranial fossa and the adjoining structures of the sella-chiasm region

1 Superior sagittal sinus (transected)
2 Tubercle of the sella turcica
3 Anterior clinoid process
4 Optic chiasm
5 Internal carotid artery
6 Terminal lamina
7 Anterior communicating artery

Bone and Wound Closure

The dura is closed with interrupted or continuous sutures. The latter are intermittently tied every 3–4 cm to prevent contraction of the dural flap. The dural elevation sutures passed through the bone are tied so as to reduce the risk of postoperative epidural hematomas. The same purpose is served by central dural sutures run through drill holes in the bone, which at the same time hold the bone flap in its position. Additional retention sutures over the bone flap may become necessary as well.

As a rule, skin closures are made with interrupted sutures.

Potential Errors and Dangers

— Overlooked blood loss due to inadequate hemostasis in the cutaneous region
— Dural injuries due to craniotomy instruments
— Injuries to the superior sagittal sinus
— Pressure lesions of the brain due to overly harsh application of brain spatulas
— Damage to optic elements
— Damage to the anterior circulus arteriosus (willisii)
— Damage to ocular nerves and olfactory nerves
— Pressure lesions of the diencephalon
— Postoperative epidural hematoma due to inadequate or slack dural elevation sutures
— Soft-tissue hematomas due to inadequate hemostasis of the skin

8 Approaches to the Central Midline Region

Transcallosal Approach to the Central Midline Region

Typical Indications for Surgery

— Tumors of the median and posterior segments of the third ventricle
— Suprapineal tumors
— Bilateral tumors of the lateral ventricle

Principal Anatomical Structures

Galea aponeurotica, superficial temporal artery (parietal branch), auriculotemporal nerve, superficial temporal vein, parietal bone, sagittal suture, middle meningeal artery and vein (frontal and parietal branches), arachnoidal granulations, superior and inferior sagittal sinus, postcentral gyrus, cingulate gyrus, superior and inferior parietal gyri, tentorium, dorsal vein of the corpus callosum, corpus callosum, commissure of the fornix. pineal body, great cerebral vein, internal cerebral vein, basal vein, posterior cerebral artery.

Positioning and Skin Incisions
(Fig. 113)

The patient is placed in a supine position, and the head is raised by 25 degrees and turned to the contralateral side by ten degrees, the anesthetist being consulted. Firm fixation is generally preferred.

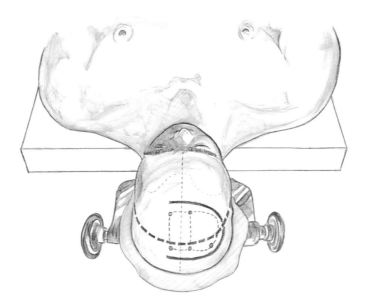

The recommended skin incision is an arcuate incision stalked toward the contralateral side and traversing the sagittal sinus; it begins 3 cm lateral to the midline, and extends to a point 2–3 cm from the temporal line. In patients with a high hairline, a U-shaped incision from ear to ear (dashed line in Fig. 113) is preferred; the skin flap is then commensurately larger, and calls for more extensive control of small hemorrhages. The galea is treated with special care in case it is needed for dural reconstruction at the end of the operation.

The skin flap is retracted out of the operative field with fishhooks or elevation sutures, while three or four heavier retention sutures are used for the same purpose on the narrow sides of the wound.

Craniotomy
(Fig. 114)

Generally, use of a single burr hole is sufficient if the bone flap is subsequently prepared with a craniotome. However, to be certain to avoid injury to the sagittal sinus, additional burr holes should be placed 1.5 cm to the side of the midline; through these holes, the space between the periosteum and the dura is distracted with a Braatz probe (inset, below right) so that the craniotome can cross the sinus plane under the protection of a watchspring probe. The Gigli saw is just as suitable for this step. Because of consistently present adhesions in the midline, the bone flap, after preparation by burr, should be cautiously detached with slender elevators. For the remainder of the operating period, the bone flap can be packed off under sterile, moist conditions. It is advisable to place the burr holes in the bone for the dural elevation sutures even before opening the dura, intervals of one centimeter at most being left between the holes. Then the dural elevation sutures are placed, but are not yet tied. Frequent small hemorrhages in the area of the sinus can be controlled advantageously with absorbable fabrics. Bipolar coagulations are rarely required. The most important landmarks are the midline, which is strongly marked at the wound margins and, after removal of the bone flap, the visible sinus region.

Fig. **113** Transcallosal approach to the central midline: positioning and incisions (overlapping arcuate incision, U-shaped incision). Black dashed lines mark the midline and the borders of the bone flap. The head is firmly fixed. The figures below show the arcuate incision crossing the midline

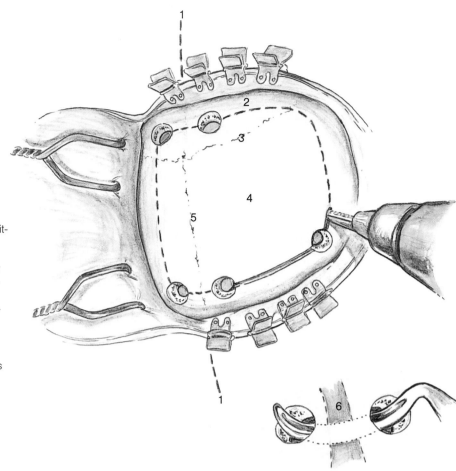

Fig. **114**   The skin flap overlapping the midline has been folded over to the contralateral side. On the bone, the coronal suture serves as an orientation aid. Burr holes are needed, above all, parasagittally to minimize the risk of injury to the superior sagittal sinus. The small figure depicts cautious retraction of the dura-invested sinus from the inner surface of the bone, using a Braatz probe. A craniotomy beyond the midline makes possible subsequent retraction of the falx and sinus to the contralateral side

1 Midline   4 Parietal bone
2 Frontal bone   5 Sagittal sinus
3 Coronal suture   6 Superior sagittal sinus

Opening the Dura
(Fig. **115**)

The dura, too, is opened by an arcuate incision with a median base. The incision is made at a distance of about one centimeter from the craniotomy border; this facilitates subsequent closure. The full craniotomy opening is utilized by tangential incisions and ensuing placement of dural retention sutures. The dural flap may be placed under a fishhook, the tension being kept low enough to safeguard the patency of the sinus and tributary veins.

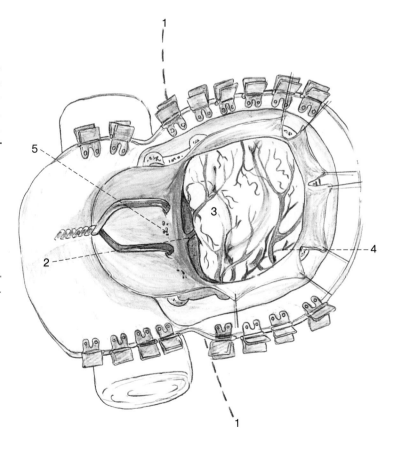

Fig. **115**   The underpadded skin flap and the dural flap are based toward the superior sagittal sinus, and have been reflected toward the midline. Retraction of the dura brings the sinus and bridging veins into view. These veins are spared if at all possible. However, the bridging vein shown in the figure requires bipolar coagulation in the vicinity of the brain. This frees access to the corpus callosum

1 Midline
2 Superior sagittal sinus and bridging vein
3 Superior frontal gyrus
4 Precentral gyrus and sulcus
5 Arachnoidal granulations

Clarification and Incision of the Corpus Callosum

(Fig. 116)

The intercerebral longitudinal fissure is entered with self-retaining spatulas. A very careful decision has to be made as to whether, and if so which, bridging veins opening into the sinus absolutely need to be coagulated and divided. A self-retaining spatula is also placed on the side of the falx, and in proportion to the bone removal, the spatula permits a slight displacement of the sinus to the contralateral side; this again will markedly improve the exposure.

When the corpus callosum, identifiable by its color and longitudinal vessels, is finally reached, it is incised longitudinally with a fine scalpel or laser. In most cases the tumor now lies directly in the field of vision. Viewed obliquely, the basal vein and the internal cerebral vein appear at the posterior border of the incision opening.

These venous conditions are shown in Figure 117.

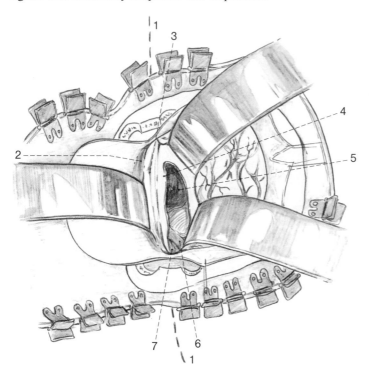

Fig. **116** The falx and the sinus have been slightly retracted to the contralateral side with a self-retaining spatula, and the brain has been retracted ipsilaterally. The corpus callosum has been incised longitudinally, so that the tumor and the deep veins are visualized

1 Midline
2 Superior sagittal sinus
3 Falx of cerebrum
4 Corpus callosum (incised)
5 Tumor
6 Right basal vein
7 Right internal cerebral vein

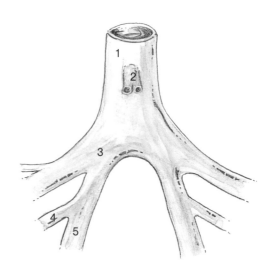

Fig. **117** Breakdown of the tributaries to the great cerebral vein (Galen's vein)

1 Great cerebral vein
2 Superior cerebellar veins
3 Basal vein
4 Occipital vein
5 Internal cerebral vein

Bone and Wound Closure

The dura is closed with interrupted sutures. If a continuous suture is used, it should be tied intermittently every 3–4 cm to avoid contraction of the dural edges.

To reduce the risk of postoperative epidural hematomas even further, two to three dural elevation sutures are run through central channels in the bone flap and are tied over the reinserted bone. Longitudinal retention sutures can reinforce the anchoring of the bone flap.

Following renewed verification of local hemostasis and possible insertion of a suction drain, the skin incision is closed with interrupted sutures.

Potential Errors and Dangers

— Overlooked blood loss due to inadequate hemostasis in the cutaneous region
— Dural injuries due to craniotomy instruments
— Sinus injuries due to craniotomy instruments
— Pressure lesions of the brain and sinus due to overly vigorous application of brain spatulas
— Too large an incision of the corpus callosum
— Lesions of deeper arteries and veins
— Pressure lesions of the basal ganglia
— Postoperative epidural hematoma due to inadequate or slack dural elevation sutures
— Soft-tissue hematoma due to inadequate hemostasis in the cutaneous region

Parietal Transventricular Approach to the Central Midline Region

Typical Indications for Surgery

- Papilloma of the choroid plexus in the lateral ventricle
- Primary and secondary tumors in the cella media region
- Arteriovenous malformations in and on the lateral ventricle

Principal Anatomical Structures

Galea aponeurotica, middle meningeal artery (parietal branch), superficial temporal vein, auriculotemporal nerve, parietal bone, squamous suture, sagittal suture, arachnoidal granulations, postcentral sulcus, lateral sulcus, angular gyrus, superior and inferior parietal gyri, supramarginal artery (from the middle cerebral artery), lateral ventricle, head and body of the caudate nucleus, choroid plexus, anterior choroidal artery, superior choroidal vein, thalamostriate vein.

Positioning and Skin Incisions
(Fig. **118**)

The patient is placed in a supine position; the head is raised 20 degrees, and may be turned to the side by 20 degrees. Alternatively, the ipsilateral shoulder can be underpadded and the head turned to the side sufficiently to position the

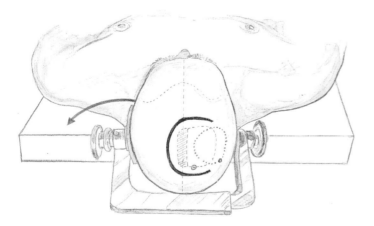

Fig. **118** Parietal transventricular approach to the central midline region: positioning and incision (arcuate incision crossing the midline). The head may either be positioned straight and elevated, or turned 60 degrees to the contralateral side; it is firmly fixed. In the figures below, the head has been turned to the contralateral side. Which position is chosen depends on the proposed craniotomy; that is to say, the head is kept straight for a craniotomy intended to go beyond the midline (black dashed line), and the head is turned for a craniotomy in the parietal bone (black dotted line)

operative field in the horizontal plane. In the former case, the surgeon proceeds from the area of the vertex; in the latter case, he or she operates from the side.

The skin flap, based in the direction of the temporal line, is curved toward the middle. It lies above the postcentral-parietal region, and may cross the midline in the presence of extensive tumors. If it does, a craniotomy going beyond the midline is planned as well. Thus, the position of the skin flap is shifted more toward the side of the operation or away from it, depending on the location of the craniotomy opening on the horizontal line.

After careful hemostasis of hemorrhages, no matter how small, the skin flap is kept out of the operative field with fishhooks or elevation sutures.

Craniotomy
(Fig. **119**)

To begin with, a burr hole is placed in the posterior part of the wound; the dura is retracted with Braatz probes, and the bone flap is prepared with a craniotome. Of course, several burr holes can be placed as well, Braatz and watchspring probes may be used, and the craniotomy can be carried out with the Gigli saw. As a rule, the bone flap is removed and packed away under moist and sterile conditions during the period of the operation. In principle, it may also be left in place on the reflected skin flap, in a permanently wet wrapping. In the next step, the holes for the dural elevation sutures should be drilled into the bone margin and the dural elevation sutures drawn in. They are not tied until the end of the operation; however, owing to their tension, epidural oozing hemorrhages can be controlled even at the start of the operation.

The most important landmark is the carefully plotted midline. In order to take advantage of the full size of the approach, 3–4 retention sutures are placed in the narrow margins of the wound.

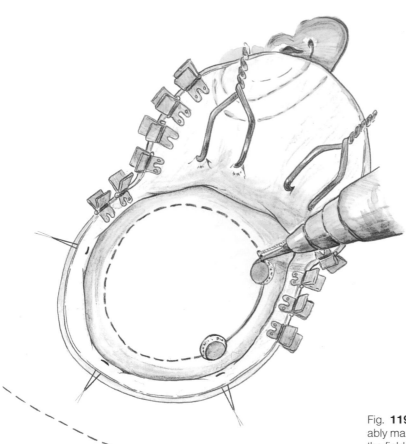

Fig. **119**   The skin flap is retracted laterally; the midline has been durably marked on the skin. The three adjacent cranial sutures do not enter the field of vision in these smaller craniotomies, but can be visualized by elevation of the galea. Thus, the marked midline and the ear serve as landmarks

Opening the Dura
(Fig. **120**)

The incision of the dura is directed laterally, and is kept at a distance of barely one centimeter from the bone margin; this facilitates the final suture of the dura. Additional radial sutures provide for full utilization of the craniotomy opening. The dural flaps are elevated by suture. The actual dural flap is kept out of the operative field with the transposed fishhook or by use of additional tension sutures.

After this, the incision site of the brain surface can be verified. On the nondominant side, use is made of the angular gyrus, and on the dominant side use is made of the area between the superior parietal and the inferior parietal gyrus, tending more toward the inferior gyrus (Fig. **120**).

Electrostimulation is also used. The procedure in the depth of the sulcus shortens the approach.

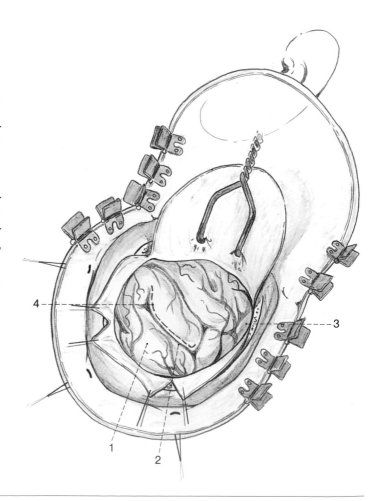

Fig. **120**   The dural incision, too, is based laterally. The incision line (red dashed line) lies in or closely behind the postcentral sulcus

1 Postcentral gyrus
2 Postcentral sulcus
3 Supramarginal gyrus
4 Incision line

Opening the Ventricle
(Fig. 121)

The advance toward the lateral ventricle is made with two microforceps, or with two slender brain spatulas. The direction can be exactly determined both preoperatively, on the basis of computed tomograms, and intraoperatively, with the aid of sonography. When the ventricle has been reached, an attempt is made to keep the opening necessary for the operative approach very small. Outlying intraventricular areas can be inspected with a small chamfered mirror or with endoscopes, so that the division in the brain and the ventricular wall can be a short procedure. At any rate, the ventricular tumors, which are already quite large in most cases, are immediately visualized, at least in part; thus, tracking the remaining parts is readily feasible.

The anatomical conditions are shown in a topside view in Figure 122. The surgeon's view is from a more lateral perspective, and covers only portions of the ventricle.

The ensuing procedure directed at the pineal region is illustrated in Figure 123, again semidiagrammatically and with the pineal gland purposely visualized. Again, the view is from above.

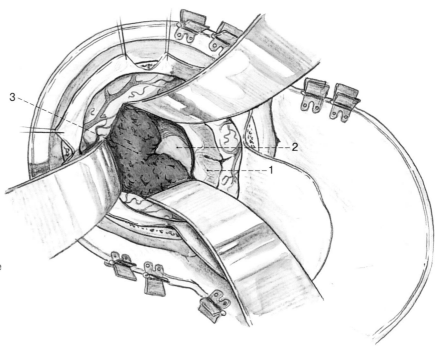

Fig. 121 The brain has been incised and the ventricle opened and developed with soft, self-retaining brain spatulas. The intraventricular tumor is brought into view

1 Parietal lobe
2 Opened right lateral ventricle
3 Tumor

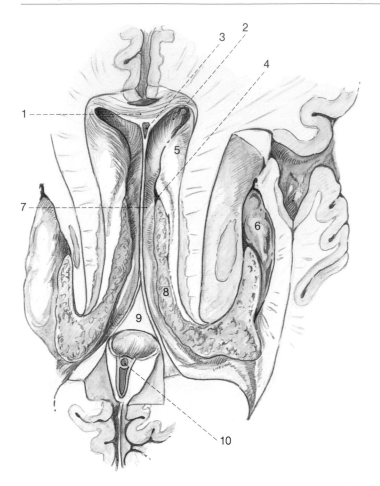

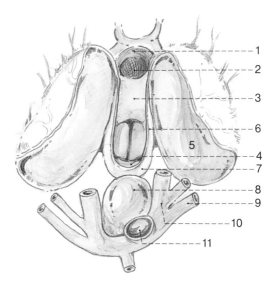

Fig. **122** Anatomy of the lateral ventricles as viewed from above. They were opened by resection of the corpus callosum, visualizing the cut borders of the genu of the corpus callosum, the septum pellucidum, and the commissure of the fornix

1	Genu of the corpus callosum	6	Hippocampus
2	Frontal horn	7	Body of the fornix
3	Cavity of the septum pellucidum	8	Choroid plexus
4	Interventricular foramen	9	Commissure of the fornix
5	Head of the caudate nucleus	10	Great cerebral vein

Fig. **123** Anatomy of pineal body and surrounding structures as viewed from above after resection of the tela of the third ventricle at the thalamic taenia and in the area of the suprapineal recess

1	Rostral commissure	7	Habenula
2	Third ventricle	8	Pineal body
3	Adhesio interthalamica	9	Basal vein
4	Commissure of the epithalamus	10	Internal cerebral vein
5	Thalamus	11	Great cerebral vein
6	Taenia thalami		(Galen's vein)

Bone and Wound Closure

The dura is closed with interrupted sutures. If a continuous suture is used, knots should be tied intermittently every 3–4 cm to prevent contraction of the dural suture. Hereafter, the dural elevation sutures that were placed immediately after the craniotomy and were passed through the bone margin are tied.

Four more centrally positioned drill holes, through which two dural elevation sutures are threaded, are made in the bone flap, and the sutures are tied at its surface. This is a preventive measure against postoperative hematomas, and also ensures adequate fixation of the bone flap in its original bed. The fixation can be reinforced with tension sutures.

After final examination of hemostasis in the subcutaneous and cutaneous regions, the operation can be concluded with interrupted sutures of the skin. If indicated, a suction drain can be inserted beneath the skin and brought out through the skin a few centimeters toward the posterior.

Potential Errors and Dangers

— Overlooked blood loss due to inadequate hemostasis in the cutaneous region
— Dural injuries due to craniotomy instruments
— Damage to functionally important brain regions due to inadequate localization prior to the brain incision
— Brain lesions due to overly vigorous application of spatulas
— Damage to deep-seated structures due to excessively large approaches
— Postoperative epidural hematoma due to inadequate or slack dural elevation sutures
— Soft-tissue hematoma due to inadequate hemostasis in the skin

9 Approaches to the Quadrigeminal and Pineal Regions

Supratentorial Approach to the Quadrigeminal and Pineal Regions

Typical Indication for Surgery

— Meningioma of the pineal region

Principal Anatomical Structures

Galea aponeurotica, occipitofrontal muscle (venter occipitalis), occipital artery and vein, greater and lesser occipital nerve, sternocleidomastoid muscle, trapezoid muscle, tendinous arch, semispinalis capitis muscle, parietal bone, occipital bone (superior squama), external occipital protuberance, lambdoid suture, sagittal suture, supreme nuchal line, occipital dipoloic vein, dura mater, transverse sinus, superior sagittal sinus, parieto-occipital sulcus, lunate sulcus, cuneus, precuneus, middle occipital artery (calcarine and parieto-occipital branches), sinus rectus, inferior sagittal sinus, great cerebral vein, superior cerebellar artery and vein, cerebral falx, tentorium, quadrigeminal lamina, pineal body.

Positioning and Skin Incision

(Fig. **124**)

The patient is placed in a sitting position and the head is firmly restrained. Forward flexing of the head has to be per-

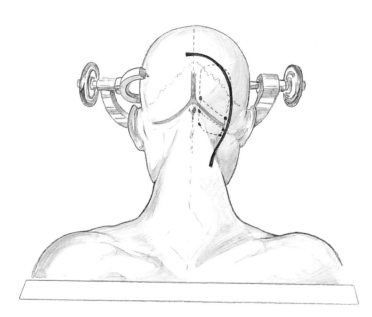

Fig. **124** Supratentorial approach to the quadrigeminal and pineal regions: positioning and incision. *Black dashed line:* the craniotomy borders. *Blue:* the two sinuses. The external occipital protuberance is palpable

formed after consultation with the anesthetist to avoid any impairment of vessels or airways.

The skin incision is in the shape of the end of a hockey stick, and begins slightly beyond the midline in the area of the lambdoid suture. It runs laterally to a point 6 cm to the side of the midline and then curves into the neck, where it ends 3 cm beside the midline, just passing the border of the trapezius muscle. Along this path it may collide with the occipital artery, but its closure does not usually cause any serious deficits. More important is the concomitant greater occipital nerve, the main trunk of which has to be spared and retracted. Beyond the tendinous arch, the incision divides the semispinalis capitis muscle at its attachment.

Craniotomy

(Fig. **125**)

With appropriate reduction of the brain volume by dehydration and removal of cerebrospinal fluid, an osteoplastic craniotomy immediately above the transverse sinus may be altogether adequate. Placement of a single drill hole and subsequent craniotome preparation of the occipital bone flap will then also suffice. The median approach extends to one centimeter short of the sagittal sinus, the leading landmarks comprising an exact outline of the midline on the scalp and the palpable external occipital protuberance.

Alternatively, either primarily or in a second step during the intracranial operation, an ensuing craniotomy can be extended beyond the transverse sinus toward the cerebellar region. Through adjacent burr holes, the dura investing the sinus is retracted from the inner periosteum, so that another bone flap can be prepared with a craniotome or Gigli saw, or this bony area can be removed with a coronal burr (inset, lower right) or with Luer forceps. The latter can be done without adverse effects by using the semitendinous muscle as a cover.

Opening the Dura

(Fig. **126**)

The dural flap is pedicled in the direction of the superior sagittal sinus. The cut border runs at a distance of barely one centimeter from the edge of the bone to facilitate the final dural suture. For full use of the craniotomy opening, radial incisions are made at the corners of the craniotomy, which are drawn outward with sutures.

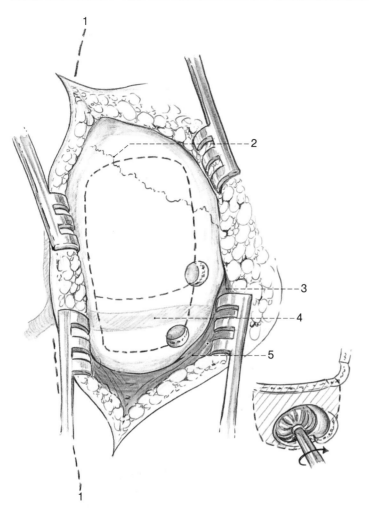

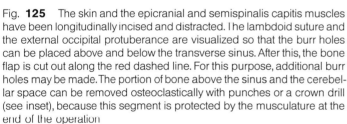

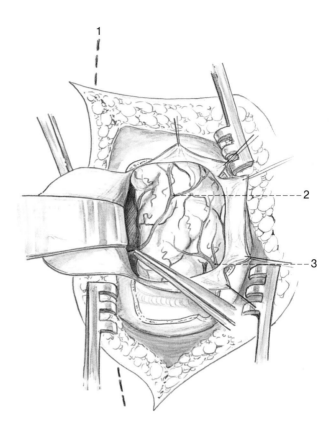

Fig. **125** The skin and the epicranial and semispinalis capitis muscles have been longitudinally incised and distracted. The lambdoid suture and the external occipital protuberance are visualized so that the burr holes can be placed above and below the transverse sinus. After this, the bone flap is cut out along the red dashed line. For this purpose, additional burr holes may be made. The portion of bone above the sinus and the cerebellar space can be removed osteoclastically with punches or a crown drill (see inset), because this segment is protected by the musculature at the end of the operation

1 Midline
2 Lambdoid suture
3 Epicranial muscle
4 Transverse sinus (presumed position)
5 Semispinalis capitis muscle

Fig. **126** The sinus and the falx have been slightly retracted to the contralateral side, so that the inside of the hemispheric fissure can be visualized. Interfering bridging veins undergo bipolar coagulation and are transected.

1 Midline
2 Occipital vein
3 Inferior cerebral vein

The portion of the occipital lobe that is now exposed has to become medially and basally mobilizable. This mobility is hindered by a few or several bridging veins between the brain surface and the two contiguous conduits. Since the operative field lies in the depth, the approach pyramid has to have a certain size at the surface, which means that one or more bridging veins have to be divided. However, the division is kept to a minimum, and an attempt is made to retain connections that are obviously of greater functional significance. The veins to be interrupted are bipolarly coagulated for a length of several millimeters, and are then divided. Special attention should be paid to keeping a sufficient distance from the sinus, so that a durable closure of the vein is achieved and no rebleeding is induced.

These important drainage channels and important local vascular supply channels are illustrated in Figure **127**.

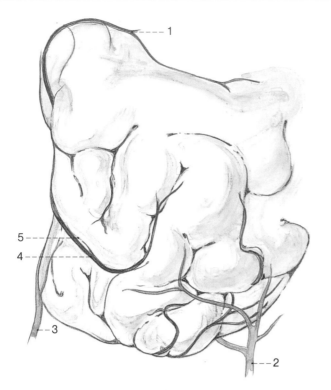

Fig. **127** Vascular courses in the region of the calcar as viewed from behind

1 Precuneate branch of the anterior cerebral arteries
2 Inferior cerebral vein
3 Internal occipital vein
4 Middle occipital artery
5 Calcarine sulcus

Exploration and Incision of the Tentorium – Exploration of the Deep Veins

(Fig. **128**)

Using a self-retaining spatula, the operator retracts the occipital lobe from the falx and then from the tentorium. As a result, the anterior and lateral border of the tentorium is gradually exposed. The incision of the tentorium is guided by the exact position of the targeted tumor. Bipolar coagulations are performed prior to the incision. The incision itself is effected in small steps, so that veins entering at the underside of the tentorium can be detected and secured in time. The posterior portions of the splenium of the corpus callosum are transected as well. Now either the tumor or the deep cerebral veins covering or accompanying it are exposed.

Understandably, the view narrows as the depth of penetration increases. This can be offset, at least in part, by slight retraction of the falx with a self-retaining spatula.

Once the craniotomy has been carried across the transverse sinus, a flap of the dura can also be opened below this conduit at any time. To avoid inadvertent injuries to the sinus, it is advisable to overlap the adjacent dural strips (Fig. **89**) and to fix them with sutures.

Bone and Wound Closure

In the majority of cases, the dura is closed with interrupted sutures. However, a continuous suture can be used as well, though this needs to be tied intermittently at intervals of 3–4 cm to prevent added dural tension.

In the next step, dural elevation sutures are placed, or the dural elevation sutures inserted into bone channels after removal of the bone flap are tied.

The bone flap, which has been packed off in a sterile, moist environment during the operation, is replaced in its bed and is fixed with dural elevation sutures, which are likewise passed through the bone. If necessary, longitudinal retention sutures can be added. Some surgeons introduce reconstruction material (plastics, lyophilized bone, drill dust from the craniotomy, etc.) into osteoclastic craniotomy areas. This type of packing is usually not absolutely necessary if there is appropriate muscle covering.

In conclusion, the hemostasis in the region of the skin flap is meticulously checked, a suction drain can be inserted, the musculature is sutured, and the required number of interrupted sutures are placed in the skin.

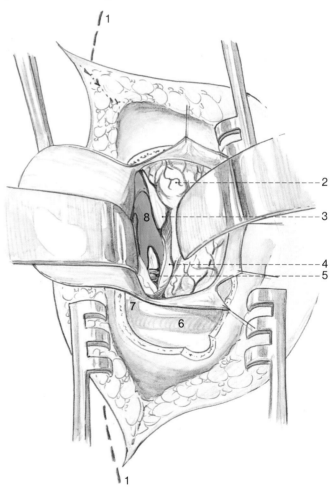

Fig. **128** The sinus-falx, on the one hand, and the occipital lobe, on the other, are held apart with self-retaining soft spatulas so that the deep cerebral veins covering the pineal body are brought into view after division of the tentorium and the posterior corpus callosum

1 Midline
2 Occipital lobe
3 Splenium of the corpus callosum
4 Tentorium of cerebellum (incised)
5 Vermis cerebelli
6 Transverse sinus
7 Superior sagittal sinus
8 Great cerebral vein (Galen's vein)

Potential Errors and Dangers

- Overlooked blood loss due to inadequate hemostasis in the cutaneous region
- Dural injuries due to craniotomy instruments
- Sinus injuries due to craniotomy instruments
- Brain damage due to excessive spatula pressure
- Division of too many veins in the craniotomy area
- Complications with infratentorial veins during the tentorial incision
- Injuries to the deep cerebral veins
- Postoperative epidural hematoma due to inadequate or slack dural elevation sutures
- Soft-tissue hematoma due to inadequate cutaneous hemostasis

Infratentorial Supracerebellar Approach to the Quadrigeminal and Pineal Regions

Typical Indications for Surgery

- Pineal gland tumors
- Malformation tumors of the pineal region and the midbrain
- Midbrain tumors
- Tumors of the cerebellar peduncles

Principal Anatomical Structures

Galea aponeurotica, trapezius muscle, splenius capitis and cervicis muscles, semispinalis capitis muscle, major and minor rectus capitis muscles, greater occipital nerve, occipital artery and vein, azygos vein of the neck, occipital bone (superior and inferior squama), external occipital protuberance, nuchal line, lambdoid suture, dura mater, transverse sinus, confluence of the sinuses, cerebellum (hemisphere), posterior inferior cerebellar artery, superior cerebellar artery, great cerebral vein, internal cerebral vein, basal vein.

Positioning and Skin Incisions

(Fig. **129**)

The patient is in the sitting position with the head firmly restrained. Some surgeons prefer to place the patient in a prone position. On this point the anesthetist ought to be consulted. For the surgeon there are no fundamental differences, as even a „reversed" anatomy is no obstacle with experience.

The skin incision corresponds to that for a typical cerebellar craniotomy, that is, it runs in a slightly undulating course over the middle of the posterior cranial fossa, but it may also be diverted to one side in the shape of a hockey stick. The incision begins at varying levels, depending on whether it is to pass below or above the transverse sinus. The upward crossing of the external occipital protuberance varies accordingly.

Great caution should be exercised with regard to emissary veins, which do not necessarily manifest themselves by active bleeding. During this phase of the operation the anesthetist should be alerted for possible air emboli. All definite and potential bone openings are immediately closed with wax, or by monopolar coagulation, or both.

In the next step, the muscles at the tendinous midline are divided with the cutting diathermy, with the fat layers possibly identifying the different muscles. Finally, strong retractors are inserted to keep the operative field open.

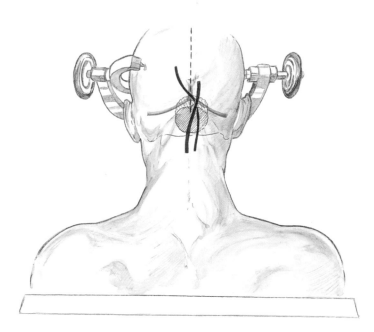

Fig. **129** Supracerebellar infratentorial approach to the quadrigeminal and pineal regions: position and incisions (S-shaped ipsilaterally and S-shaped from the contralateral side). The customary craniotomy is identified by light shading, and a possible enlargement beyond the transverse sinus by heavy shading. The midline and the typical course of the sinus (blue) are marked. The head is firmly restrained. Represented in the figures below is the incision from the contralateral side

Craniotomy

(Fig. **130**)

A burr hole is placed clearly beside the midline and at least two centimeters below the plane of the external occipital protuberance, that is, the plane of the transverse sinus. The craniotomy opening can be enlarged with Luer forceps and punches; use of a large coronal burr in the drill shank has given good results. Dural injuries due to this cutter head are rare; it is considerably more efficient than punches, and greatly eases the effort required by a surgeon who is prepared for a microscopic operation. With the burr it is also possible to pass beyond the generally readily visible area of the confluence of sinuses and the adjoining transverse sinus. Small veins that usually course in emissaries can be secured bipolarly without difficulty.

Familiarity of the surgeon with the relations between the insertion of the nuchal muscles and the external occipital protuberance to the subjacent sinuses, including their confluence, is a prerequisite (Fig. **131**).

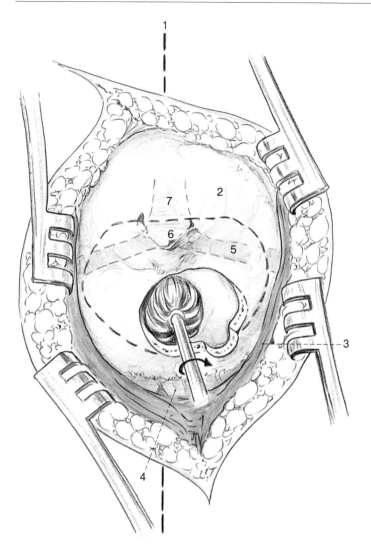

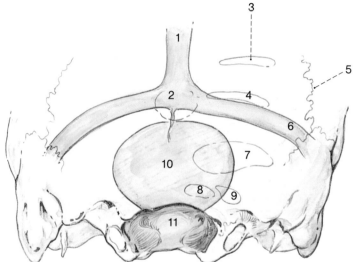

Fig. **130** The superior and inferior squamae of the occipital bone have been exposed; the periosteum is retracted. After placement of an infratentorial burr hole, the craniotomy can be carried out with punches or a crown drill inside the red dashed line

1 Midline
2 Occipital bone
3 Semispinalis capitis muscle (incised)
4 Rectus capitis posterior minor muscle
5 Transverse sinus (presumed course)
6 External occipital protuberance
7 Superior sagittal sinus (presumed course)

Fig. **131** Involved anatomical structures as viewed from behind and below

1 Superior sagittal sinus
2 Confluence of the sinuses and external occipital protuberance
3 Insertion of the occipitofrontal muscle
4 Insertion of the trapezius muscle
5 Lambdoid suture
6 Transverse sinus
7 Insertion of the semispinalis capitis muscle
8 Insertion of the rectus capitis posterior minor muscle
9 Insertion of the rectus capitis posterior major muscle
10 Craniotomy in the occipital bone (inferior squama)
11 Great foramen

Opening the Dura
(Fig. 132)

Analogously to the typical craniotomy to the cerebellum, a Y-shaped incision is made in the dura. The upper portions of the incision extend to the transverse sinus, but are made in small steps only, because of possible lacunae. The occipital sinus is more strongly developed only in rare cases. However, at times the cerebellar dura shows a reticular sinus penetration, so that hemostasis may present serious difficulties.

The arachnoid is left intact at first, provided this is not precluded by adhesions. It is not opened until after the dural incision, and then only in the immediate area of the approach.

After this, portions of the cerebellar hemisphere, the uvula, and the cerebellar tonsillae, as well as the local vessels, are visualized. The corresponding arteries are shown in Figure 133.

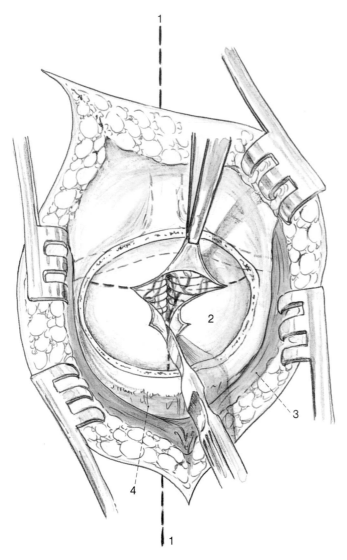

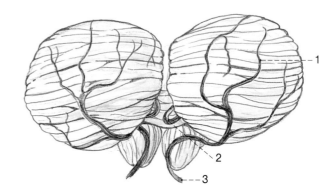

Fig. **132** A Y-shaped incision is made in the dura; in most cases, the arachnoid can be spared to begin with. Less commonly, the occipital sinus becomes a source of bleeding, the cerebellar falx hardly forming a barrier

1 Midline
2 Dura mater (incised)
3 Semispinalis capitis muscle (incised)
4 Rectus capitis posterior minor muscle

Fig. **133** Overview of the arteries of the posterior cerebellar surface

1 Hemispheric branches of posterior inferior cerebellar artery
2 Vermis branches of posterior inferior cerebellar artery
3 Posterior inferior cerebellar artery

Dissection of the Cerebellum and Exposure of the Veins

(Fig. 134)

In the next dissection step, the space between the cerebellar surface and the underside of the tentorium is entered. A varying number of bridging veins is found between the cerebellum and the underside of the tentorium. Whether these veins can be spared has to be decided in each individual case. If they need to be divided, bipolar coagulation should be performed at a sufficient distance from the tentorium and the cerebellum, so that rebleeding may be avoided.

With the use of a self-retaining retractor, the cerebellum is displaced inferiorly, so that the deep veins and accompanying adhesions are brought into view.

Subsequently, the actual tumor is exposed.

Bone and Wound Closure

The dura can be closed with interrupted or continuous sutures. The latter are intermittently tied every 3–4 cm. Dural elevation sutures are seldom required, because fairly solid adhesions exist between the cerebellar dura and the remaining portion of the occipital bone.

Reconstruction materials (plastics, lyophilized bone, burr material from the craniotomy) can be packed into the craniotomy gap. However, because of the good cover provided by the nuchal musculature, this type of packing often seems unnecessary.

Potential Errors and Dangers

— Overlooked blood loss due to inadequate cutaneous hemostasis
— Air embolism due to overlooked opening of emissaries and lack of control by the anesthetist
— Dural injuries due to craniotomy instruments
— Sinus injuries due to craniotomy instruments
— Cerebellar lesions due to excessive spatula pressure
— Laceration of bridging veins
— Injuries to deep cerebral veins
— Postoperative hematomas on both sides of the dura and in the soft tissues, due to reopening of previously stopped sources of bleeding

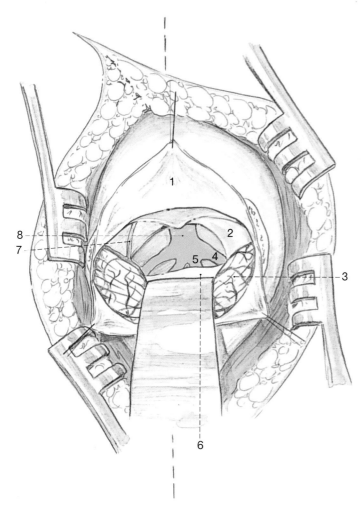

Fig. **134** Following closure of bridging veins between the cerebellum and the tentorium the quadrigeminal region can be explored with soft, self-retaining spatulas

1 Elevated dura mater
2 Tentorium with tentorial border
3 Right hemisphere of the cerebellum
4 Right basal vein
5 Right internal cerebral vein
6 Culmen of the cerebellar vermis
7 Spared bridging vein between the cerebellum and the tentorium
8 Great cerebral vein (Galen's vein)

10 Approaches to the Posterior Cranial Fossa

Median Approach to the Posterior Cranial Fossa

Typical Indications for Surgery

— Midline tumors of the posterior cranial fossa
— Tumors in the fourth ventricle
— Malformations
— Parasites
— Angiomas
— Inflammatory alterations

Principal Anatomical Structures

External occipital protuberance, spinous process of the axis, azygos vein of the neck, cutaneous branches and dorsal branch of cervical nerves 3, 4, and 5, trapezius muscle, semispinalis capitis muscle, splenius capitis muscle, splenius cervicis muscle, sternocleidomastoid muscle, occipital squama, posterior arch of atlas, superior and inferior nuchal line, atlanto-occipital membrane, dura mater, arachnoid, inferior cerebellar veins, posterior inferior cerebellar artery (PICA), cerebellar tonsillae, vermis cerebelli, cerebellar hemispheres.

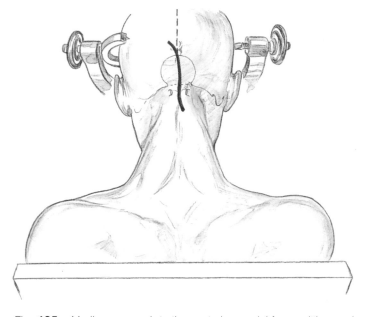

Fig. **135**   Median approach to the posterior cranial fossa: sitting position, with firmly fixed head. The craniotomy border and the resected atlantal arch are marked. The sitting position is represented in the figures below

Positioning and Skin Incisions

(Figs. **135, 136**)

The operation can be performed in the prone or the sitting position. In the prone position, there is a greater tendency for venous hemorrhages to occur; in the sitting position, there is a greater risk of air embolism. In both positions, a central venous catheter is required. The strongly fixed head of the seated patient is flexed forward slightly; that is, the chin moves toward the jugular fossa. The flexion should not be excessive, however, particularly in the presence of degenerative changes of the cervical spine. In the recumbent position, the head is slightly tilted downward; here again, the flexion should be moderate. An S-shaped incision is made in the midline; beginning at the external occipital protuberance, it extends as far as the processus spinalis epistrophei. The fascia and the musculature are divided in the midline and retracted laterally (Fig. **137**). A muscle stump is left in place at the superior nuchal line. This facilitates approximation of the musculature during wound closure. Bleeding from the bone is controlled with bone wax, and hemorrhages at the occipital membrane are arrested by coagulation.

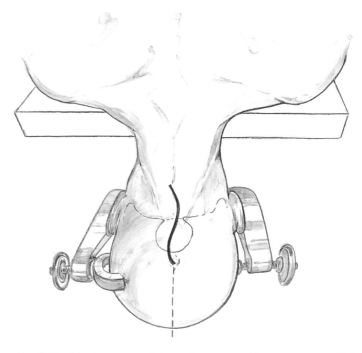

Fig. **136**   Median approach to posterior cranial fossa: prone position with the head firmly fixed. The craniotomy border is marked

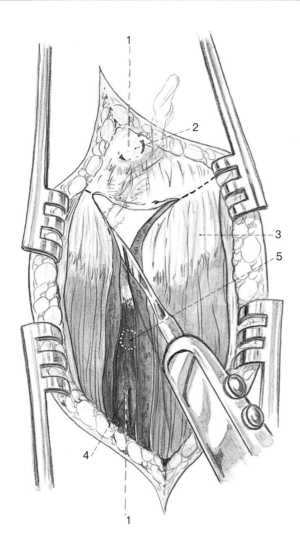

Fig. **137** A mildly S-shaped incision has been made in the skin and fatty tissue. The musculature is divided in the tendinous midline, and is notched at its insertion

1 Midline
2 External occipital protuberance
3 Semispinalis capitis muscle
4 Rectus capitis posterior minor muscle
5 Palpable arch of the atlas

Fig. **138** The musculature has been retracted to the sides and as far as the border of the great foramen, so that the posterior cranial fossa can be opened osteoclastically from one burr hole, using punches or the crown drill

1 Midline
2 External occipital protuberance
3 Trapezius and semispinalis capitis muscles
4 Bone still to be removed
5 Rectus capitis posterior minor muscle

Craniotomy
(Fig. **138**)

One burr hole each is placed in paramedian position in the occipital squama over the cerebellar hemispheres. A distance of at least 2 cm from the sinus should be maintained. Occasionally, the dura over the cerebellar hemispheres is very thin and fragile; this requires careful attention during the osteoclastic craniectomy. Using bone forceps of all kinds (curved, angulated, straight, etc.), the bone is bilaterally removed down to the transverse sinus and very close to the confluence of sinuses. In the presence of very strong occipital squamae, particularly in the confluence area, the bone can be thinned with burrs. The transverse sinus has to be exposed as far as its inferior border, as there would otherwise not be sufficient visualization or space for an operative procedure in the depth. In case of intracranial pressure or tumors extending to C1 or C2, a partial resection of the atlantal arch has to be carried out (Fig. **139**). It should be borne in mind that the vertebral arteries enter the area of the great foramen at the superior border of the lateral atlantal arch.

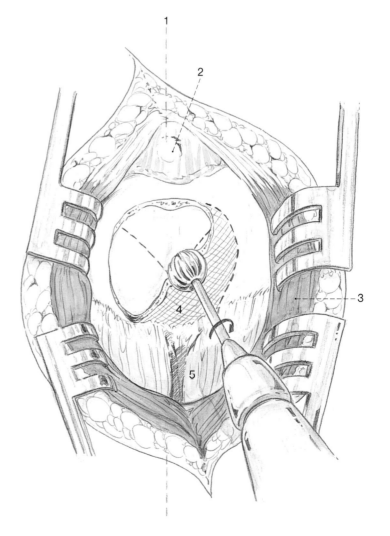

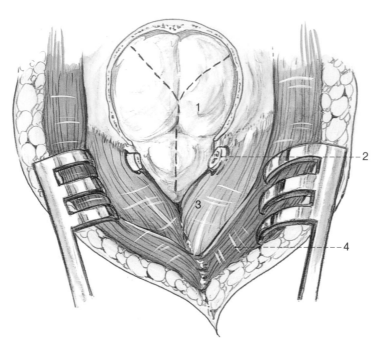

Fig. **139** Osteoclastic cerebellar craniotomy, with removal of the atlantal arch. This allows the Y-shaped dural incision to be extended to a point below the cerebellar tonsils

1 Dura mater over the cerebellar hemispheres and cerebellar tonsils
2 Stumps of the atlantal arch
3 Rectus capitis posterior major muscle
4 Semispinalis capitis and trapezius muscles

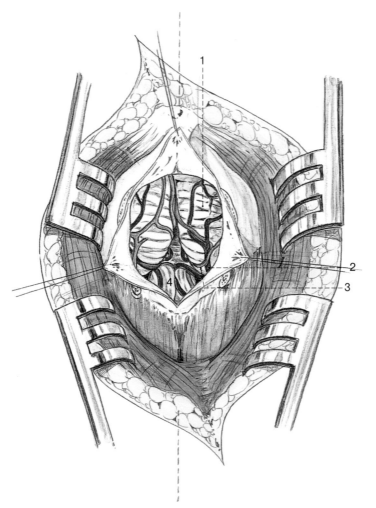

Opening the Dura
(Fig. 140)

As a general rule, the dura over the midline of the posterior cranial fossa is opened by a Y-shaped incision, the two arms extending to the transverse sinus, and the vertical leg of the Y heading in the cervical direction. The dura should always be opened as far as C1–C2 to allow easy inspection of the cerebellar tonsillae. The occipital sinus, which develops with considerable variations, requires a double ligature in all cases. After the twofold ligation of the occipital sinus, it is transected with scissors. Spatulas are inserted from each side to protect subjacent structures. The dura can now be opened in a cervical direction by a paramedian incision. Not uncommonly, the arachnoid is left in place and has to be opened with a sharp hook. Major arachnoid resections ought to be avoided (scar formation).

Details of the anatomy are shown in Figure **141**.

Fig. **140** After the Y-shaped opening of the dura and retraction of the arachnoid the cerebellar hemispheres, the vermis and tonsils are exposed, with the vessels coursing superiorly

1 Cerebellar hemisphere
2 Posterior inferior cerebellar artery and branches
3 Inferior vein of cerebellar hemisphere
4 Cerebellar tonsil

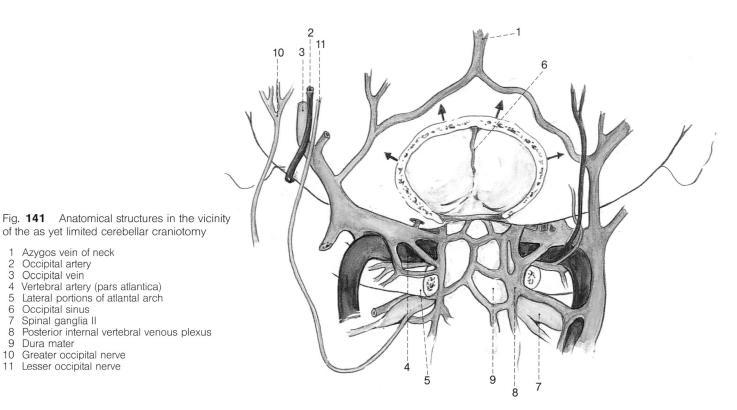

Fig. **141** Anatomical structures in the vicinity of the as yet limited cerebellar craniotomy

 1 Azygos vein of neck
 2 Occipital artery
 3 Occipital vein
 4 Vertebral artery (pars atlantica)
 5 Lateral portions of atlantal arch
 6 Occipital sinus
 7 Spinal ganglia II
 8 Posterior internal vertebral venous plexus
 9 Dura mater
10 Greater occipital nerve
11 Lesser occipital nerve

Dural and Wound Closure

Watertight suture of the dura is required in order to prevent cerebrospinal fluid fistulas. If there is not enough endogenous dura available for closure, a pedicled muscle-fascia flap, or a free fascia lata reconstruction, is recommended. Heterologous materials or adhesives are best avoided. The muscles are gently approximated and sutured to the residual muscle stump in the area of the nuchal line. The subcutis should be tightly closed. The skin should be closed without excessive suture traction because necroses may otherwise develop in the nuchal region. The use of suction drains near the sinus is not advisable.

Potential Errors and Dangers

— Overlooked blood loss at the cut borders of the skin or from bone margins
— Injuries to the dura or the cerebellar cortex due to craniotomy instruments
— Pressure lesions of the cerebellum due to improper or hasty use of brain spatulas
— Injury to a venous conduit
— Injuries to bridging veins
— Postoperative hemorrhages from inadequately secured vessels at the cerebellar surface
— Epidural hemorrhages due to inadequate dural elevation sutures or from soft tissues
— Soft-tissue hematomas

Paramedian Unilateral Approach to the Posterior Cranial Fossa

Typical Indications for Surgery

— Hemispheric tumors of the cerebellum
— Angiomas
— Hemorrhages
— Space-occupying infarcted areas of the cerebellar hemisphere
— Malformations
— Inflammatory processes

Principal Anatomical Structures

Occipitofrontal muscle (venter occipitalis), greater occipital artery and vein, greater occipital nerve, lesser occipital nerve, trapezius muscle, sternocleidomastoid muscle, occipital squama, dura mater, vertebral artery.

Positioning and Skin Incisions

(Fig. 142)

For this approach, too, both the sitting and the recumbent position are possible. In both cases, the head is firmly fixed and rotated about 30 degrees toward the side of the lesion.

Caution has to be exercised in turning and tilting the restrained head when degenerative changes of the spinal column are present. Either an S-shaped or a straight skin incision may be chosen. The greater occipital nerve and the accompanying artery and vein sometimes cannot be spared in this approach.

Incision of Soft Tissues

(Fig. 143)

As far as possible, the musculature is opened along the natural borders of adjoining muscles. Electrocautery division is required in the deeper layers. Vessels and nerves at this level are shown in Figure 144.

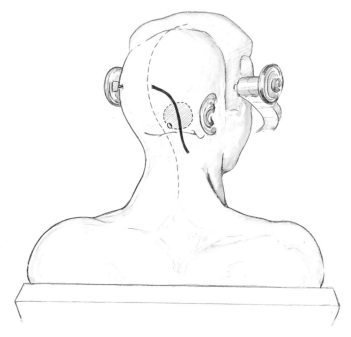

Fig. **142** Right-sided paramedian approach to the posterior cranial fossa: positioning and incision. The head is firmly fixed. *Shading:* the craniotomy defect

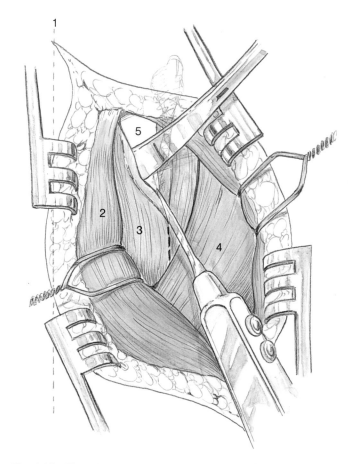

Fig. **143** The skin incision is followed by layered electrocautery division of the investing musculature

1 Midline
2 Trapezius muscle (incised)
3 Semispinalis capitis muscle (incised)
4 Splenius capitis muscle
5 Occipital bone (squama)

Craniotomy
(Fig. 145)

After placement of a burr hole in the occipital squama, the bone defect is osteoclastically expanded to the necessary size with Luer forceps. The dura over the cerebellar hemisphere is often adherent to the bone, and has to be carefully retracted. Hemorrhages from the bone are controlled with bone wax.

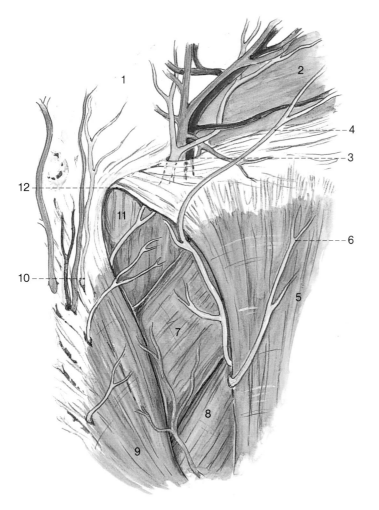

Fig. **144** Right-sided anatomical structures lateral to the craniocervical region

1 Occipital bone (squama)
2 Occipitofrontal muscle (venter occipitalis)
3 Occipital artery and vein, and greater occipital nerve
4 Lesser occipital nerve
5 Sternocleidomastoid muscle
6 Great auricular nerve
7 Splenius capitis muscle
8 Splenius cervicis muscle
9 Trapezius muscle
10 Third occipital nerve
11 Semispinalis capitis muscle
12 Tendinous arch between the sternocleidomastoid and trapezius muscles

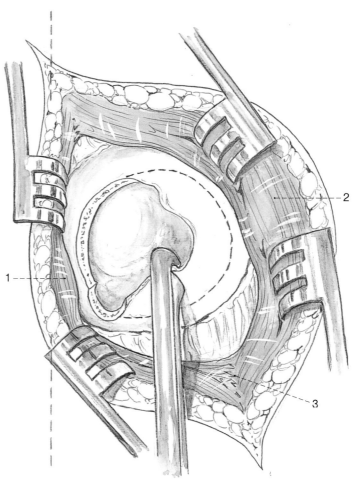

Fig. **145** The muscles are retracted; the periosteum has been moved out of the way. After placement of a burr hole, the osteoclastic craniotomy can be carried out in the area defined by dashed lines, using punches or the crown drill.

1 Semispinalis capitis muscle
2 Trapezius muscle
3 Splenius capitis muscle

Opening the Dura

(Fig. 146)

The dura is opened by a cruciform, stellate, or arcuate incision; any resultant dural cusps are elevated by suture. When the dura is elevated from the cerebellar surface, attention has to be paid to bridging veins and adhesions. The process in the hemisphere is localized intraoperatively by ultrasound. Displacements of cerebellar nuclei by space-occupying processes are shown in Figure 147.

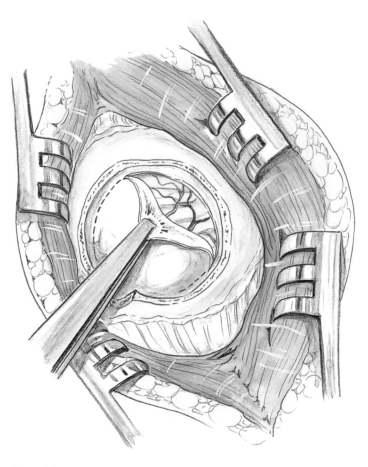

Fig. **146** After completion of the osteoclastic craniotomy, the dura is opened, with a basal pedicle, along the dashed line. Below it, the right cerebellar hemisphere is visualized

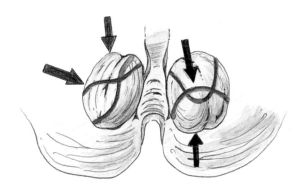

Fig. **147** Displacements and deformities of the dentate nucleus – depending on the direction of pressure – due to a space-occupying mass

Dural and Wound Closure

The dura is closed with interrupted sutures. Elevation sutures of the dura are placed prior to closure of the dura and are tied after the closure. Covering of the bone gap created by the osteoclastic craniotomy is not necessary. The wound is closed in layers.

Potential Errors and Dangers

— Overlooked blood loss during the operation from skin, muscle and/or bone
— Injuries of the dura or cerebellar cortex due to craniotomy instruments
— Pressure lesions of the cerebellum due to improper or hasty procedure in applying the brain spatula
— Postoperative hemorrhages from the cerebellar surface, from bridging veins, or due to inadequate dural elevation sutures
— Epidural hemorrhages from the dura or soft tissues

Retrosigmoid (Retroauricular) Approach to the Posterior Cranial Fossa

Typical Indications for Surgery

- Space-occupying processes in the cerebellopontine angle
- Arteriovenous malformations in the cerebellopontine angle
- Aneurysms in the area of the cerebellopontine angle
- Compression syndromes of cranial nerves (5, 7, 8, 9, 10)
- Inflammatory processes in the area of the cerebellopontine angle

Principal Anatomical Structures

Helix, external occipital protuberance, superior nuchal line, sternocleidomastoid muscle, splenius capitis muscle, lesser occipital nerve (auricular branches), great auricular nerve, posterior auricular nerve, mastoid process, venous emissary, sigmoid sinus, transverse sinus, dura mater.

Positioning and Skin Incision

(Fig. **148**)

With the patient seated, the restrained head has to be turned to the side of the lesion by about 30 degrees. It is important for the chin to be flexed slightly toward the jugular fossa. A slightly S-shaped skin incision is performed.

In the recumbent position, the restrained head has to be turned away from the lesion by about 30 to 40 degrees. In this case, too, an S-shaped incision is preferred. The auricle is retracted with adhesive tape (or a suture).

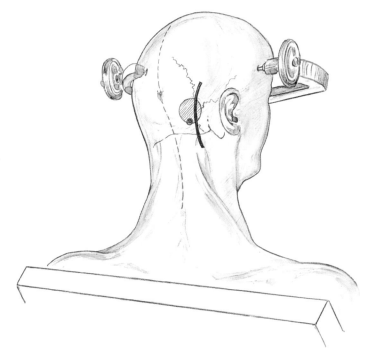

Fig. **148** Rectosigmoid approach to the cerebellopontine angle: positioning and incision. *Black shading:* the craniotomy defect to be produced. Palpable adjacent structures include the external occipital protuberance and the mastoid

Incision of Soft Tissues and Craniotomy
(Fig. **149**)

After being incised, the fasciae and muscles are retracted with a raspatory and held off with a retractor. After placing a burr hole, the bone is ablated osteoclastically with Luer forceps (or a drilling head). The bone has to be removed down to the inferior border of the transverse sinus and as far as the border of the sigmoid sinus. In addition, the angle at which the transverse sinus opens into the sigmoid sinus has to be exposed. Venous hemorrhages into the bone are controlled with bone wax, and emissaries are likewise sealed. Opened, pneumatized mastoid cells should be roofed over with fascia by the appropriate technique.

Suggestions for optimal placement of burr holes are presented in Figure **150**. Figure **151** illustrates the anatomical relations between the craniotomy opening and the sinus.

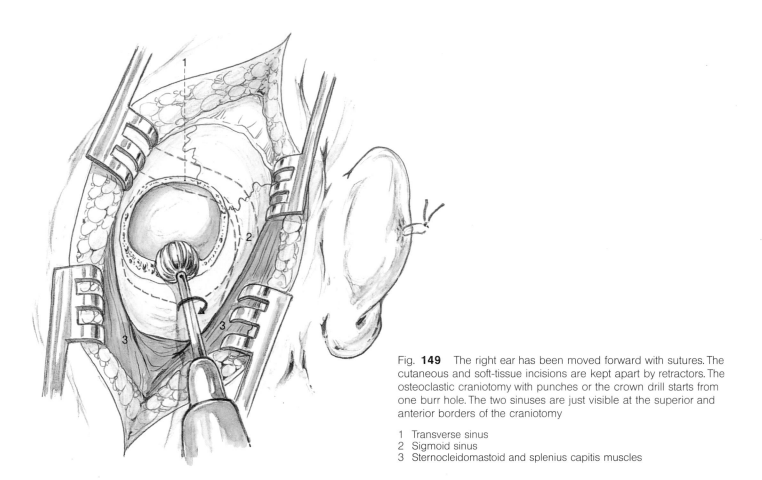

Fig. **149** The right ear has been moved forward with sutures. The cutaneous and soft-tissue incisions are kept apart by retractors. The osteoclastic craniotomy with punches or the crown drill starts from one burr hole. The two sinuses are just visible at the superior and anterior borders of the craniotomy

1 Transverse sinus
2 Sigmoid sinus
3 Sternocleidomastoid and splenius capitis muscles

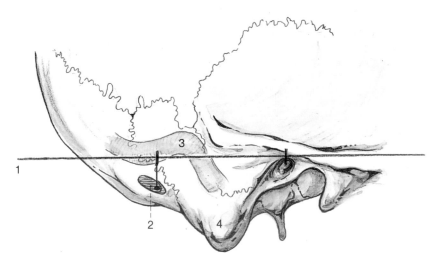

Fig. **150** Planning for optimal localization of the burr hole for retrosigmoid osteoclastic craniotomy

1 Frankfurt horizontal plane, with the designated distance behind the center of the external acoustic meatus: 50 mm in males, 45–50 mm in females; the optimal position of the burr hole is 11.5 mm below this line
2 Burr hole
3 Sigmoid sinus
4 Mastoid

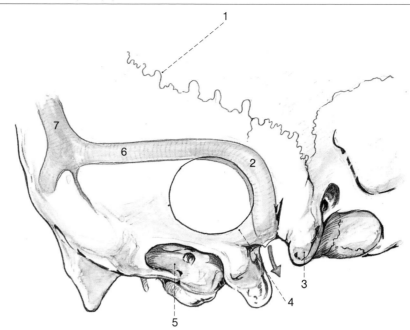

Fig. **151** The anatomical relations between the sinuses and the retrosigmoid craniotomy

1 Lambdoid suture
2 Sigmoid sinus
3 Mastoid
4 Craniotomy opening
5 Great foramen
6 Transverse sinus
7 Superior sagittal sinus

Incision of Dura

(Fig. **152**)

The dura is opened by an arcuate incision, with the stalk directed toward the midline. Still to be added are one or two auxiliary incisions toward the sinuses; the resulting dural flap is elevated by a suture. The pedicled dural flap, as a partial covering of the cerebellum, may serve for spatula support. Any bridging veins are coagulated and divided.

In this way, the cerebellopontine angle is brought into view. Anatomical details are shown in Figures **153** and **154**.

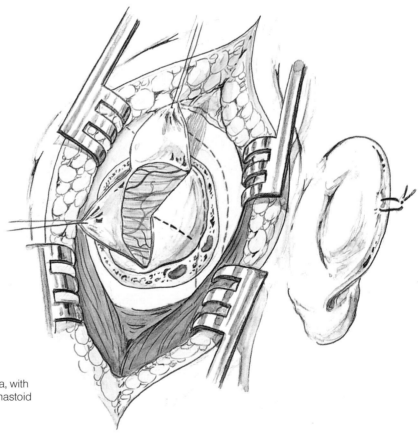

Fig. **152** A K-shaped incision is made in the exposed dura, with the two arms of the K directed toward the sinuses. Opened mastoid cells are immediately covered over with wax (green)

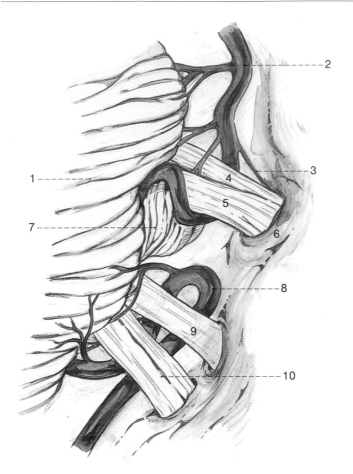

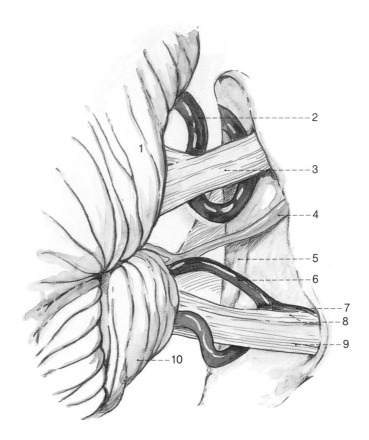

Fig. **153** Nerves and arteries in the cerebellopontine angle, as seen by the surgeon

1 Cerebellum (hemisphere)
2 Anterior inferior cerebellar artery (AICA)
3 Labyrinthine artery
4 Facial nerve
5 Vestibulocochlear nerve
6 Internal acoustic pore
7 Cerebellar flocculus
8 Posterior inferior cerebellar artery (PICA)
9 Glossopharyngeal nerve
10 Vagus nerve

Fig. **154** Retrosigmoid approach in the area of the trigeminal nerve in vascular compression syndrome: relations between the trigeminal nerve, brain stem, and local vessels (highly variable)

1 Cerebellum
2 Superior cerebellar artery
3 Trigeminal nerve
4 Petrosal vein
5 Abducens nerve
6 Anterior inferior cerebellar artery (AICA)
7 Labyrinthine artery
8 Facial nerve
9 Statoacoustic nerve
10 Cerebellar flocculus

Dural and Wound Closure

Interrupted sutures are used for a watertight closure of the dura. In the absence of sufficient indigenous dura, autologous materials for closure of the dura are preferred. The musculature is approximated. Subcutis and cutis are sutured. The application of suction drains in the proximity of the sinus or in the presence of open cerebrospinal fluid spaces is inadvisable.

Potential Errors and Dangers

— Faulty positioning of the patient
— Faulty rotation of the restrained head
— Overlooked hemorrhages from skin, muscle, or bone during the operation
— Air embolism over veins or emissaries, particularly with the patient in the sitting position
— Absence of a central venous catheter
— Injuries to the dura or the cerebellar cortex due to craniotomy instruments
— Pressure lesions of the cerebellum or brain stem due to improper or hasty use of the brain spatula
— Postoperative hemorrhages from the cerebellar surface, from bridging veins, or due to inadequate dural elevation sutures
— Epidural hemorrhages from the dura or soft tissues

Median Suboccipital Approach to the Posterior Cranial Fossa

Typical Indications for Surgery

− Processes in the great foramen
− Tractotomy and partial nucleotomy
− Angiomas
− Aneurysms
− Inflammatory processes
− Malformations (Arnold-Chiari, basilar impression)

Principal Anatomical Structures

External occipital protuberance, azygos vein of the neck, cutaneous branches and dorsal branch of the third, fourth and fifth cervical nerves, trapezius muscle, semispinalis capitis muscle, splenius capitis and cervicis muscles, occipital squama, posterior arch of atlas, vertebral artery, spinous process of the axis, atlanto-occipital membrane, dura mater of the cerebellum and spinal cord, arachnoid, posterior inferior cerebellar artery (PICA).

Positioning and Skin Incision
(Fig. 155)

Both the sitting and the recumbent position are possible. The head should be firmly fixed. In the sitting position, the chin should be moderately inclined toward the jugular fossa. The recumbent patient's head should be tilted slightly downward. The skin incision is mildly S-shaped, and reaches from the external occipital protuberance to at least the spinous process of the epistropheus (axis).

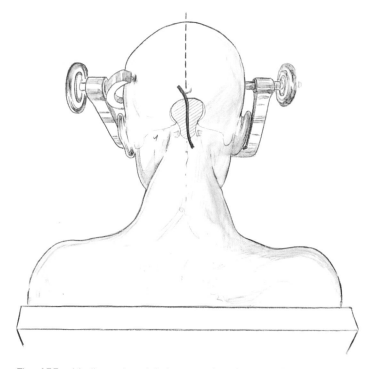

Fig. **155**　Median suboccipital approach to the posterior cranial fossa: positioning and incision. *Black:* the craniotomy defect and the resected atlantal arch. Palpable adjacent structures include the external occipital protuberance and the two mastoid processes. The head is firmly fixed

Incision of Soft Tissues
(Fig. 156)

The musculature is divided in the middle and from its attachment at the atlantal arch and the spinous process of the epistropheus, and retracted. Associated venous hemorrhages are immediately controlled. In the sitting position, air embolisms frequently develop in this phase of the dissection. About 2 cm below the superior nuchal line, the musculature is transected; the remaining muscular bulge on the occiput is needed for the subsequent wound closure.

Craniotomy and Resection of the Atlas
(Fig. 157)

Following paramedian placement of burr holes, an osteoclastic craniectomy is performed with Luer forceps. The great foramen is opened; the partial resection of the atlantal arch should extend laterally on both sides. Attention should be paid to the bilateral entry of the vertebral artery (Fig. **158**) at the lateral superior margin of the atlantal arch. Hemorrhages from the bone have to be stopped with wax.

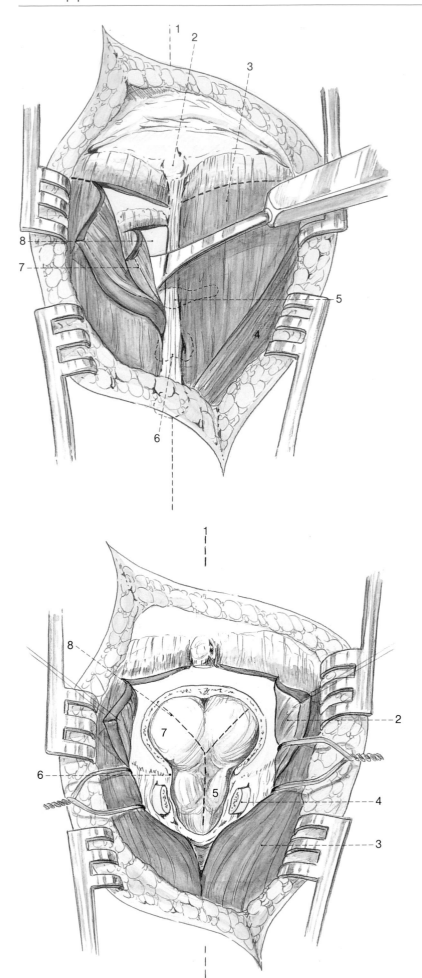

Fig. **156** Incised skin and adipose tissue are retracted. After being longitudinally incised, the muscles and periosteum are retracted from the bone

1 Midline
2 External occipital protuberance
3 Semispinalis capitis muscle
4 Splenius capitis muscle
5 Atlantal arch
6 Spinous process of the epistropheus
7 Rectus capitis posterior minor muscle
8 Occipital bone (inferior squama)

Fig. **157** The osteoclastic craniotomy over the cerebellum and resection of the atlantal arch have been carried out.
Red dashes: the Y-shaped incision of the dura

1 Midline
2 Rectus capitis posterior minor muscle
3 Semispinalis capitis muscle
4 Stumps of the resected atlantal arch
5 Cerebellar tonsils (covered by dura)
6 Posterior atlanto-occipital membrane
7 Cerebellar hemispheres (covered by dura)
8 Dural incision line (Y-shaped)

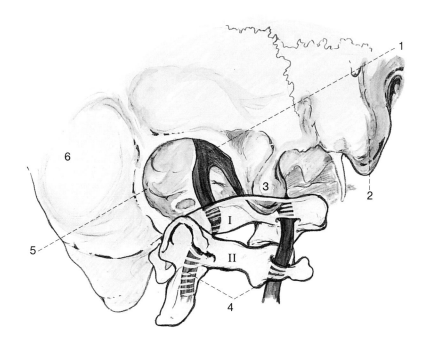

Fig. **158** Anatomical relations between the great foramen and vertebral arteries

1 Basilar artery
2 Mastoid process
3 Occipital condyle
4 Vertebral arteries
5 Great foramen
6 Occipital bone

Opening of Dura
(Fig. **159**)

A Y-shaped incision is made in the dura over the midline of the posterior cranial fossa, with the vertical leg of the Y extending in a caudal direction near the midline. To perform a tractotomy, the dura has to be opened further in a lateral direction. In addition, the cervical roots of segment C2 have to be visualized during the tractotomy. The arachnoid usually remains intact after opening of the dura. The arachnoid then has to be opened with a sharp hook or with scissors; it should not be removed (scar formation).

When opening the dura and the arachnoid, the course of the posterior inferior cerebellar artery (PICA) needs to be carefully observed (Fig. **160**).

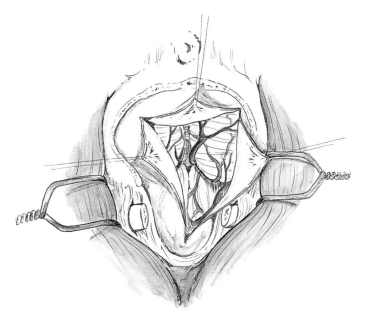

Fig. **159** Y-shaped opening of the dura. The cerebellar hemispheres and the cerebellar tonsils and overlying vessels are visualized. The cerebellomedullary cistern appears in the lowermost incision angle

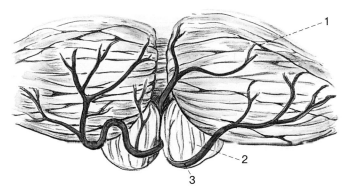

Fig. **160** Common course of posterior inferior cerebellar artery in the area of the cerebellar hemispheres and tonsils

1 Horizontal fissure of the cerebellum
2 Cerebellar tonsil
3 Posterior inferior cerebellar artery (PICA) and branches

Dural and Wound Closure

Watertight suture of the dura is required to avoid dural fistulas. Homologous or autologous materials are used for dural closure. The musculature is approximated under moderate traction, and is sutured in the area of the superior nuchal line to the muscle stump remaining. When the subcutis has been tightly sutured, the skin is closed under moderate suture traction so that subsequent skin necroses can be averted.

Potential Errors and Dangers

— Overlooked blood loss from the cut borders of the skin, the musculature, and the bone margins during the operation
— Air embolism over veins and emissaries, particularly in the sitting position
— Lack of central venous catheter
— Injuries of the dura or cerebellar cortex due to the craniotome
— Injuries of the vertebral arteries during partial resection of the atlantal arch
— Pressure lesions of the cerebellum due to improper or hasty application of brain spatulas
— Postoperative hemorrhages from the cerebellar surface, from bridging veins, or due to inadequate dural elevation sutures
— Cerebrospinal fluid fistula
— Soft-tissue hematomas

Paramedian Suboccipital Approach to the Posterior Cranial Fossa

Typical Indications for Surgery

— Tumors of the lateral brain stem
— Aneurysms of the posterior inferior cerebellar artery (PICA)
— Aneurysms of the vertebral artery
— Angiomas

Principal Anatomical Structures

External occipital protuberance, superior nuchal line, greater occipital artery and vein, trapezius muscle, semispinalis capitis muscle, splenius capitis muscle, sternocleidomastoid muscle (posterior border), occipital squama, arch of the atlas (pars lateralis), vertebral artery, atlanto-occipital membrane, dura mater, arachnoid, posterior inferior cerebellar artery (PICA), ninth, tenth and eleventh nerves; brain stem.

Positioning and Skin Incisions
(Figs. **161**, **162**)

In the sitting position, the firmly fixed head is turned about 30 degrees toward the lesion. With the patient lying down, the occipital squama and the skin incision to be made are at the highest points of the immobilized head. The skin incisions are lightly S-shaped and have to pass over the level of the atlantal arch.

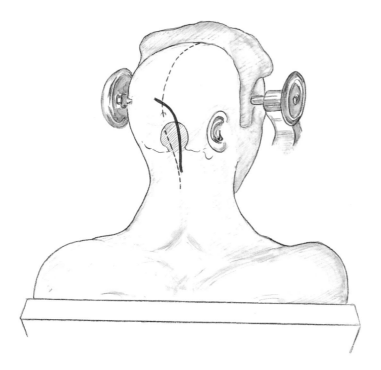

Fig. **161** Paramedian suboccipital approach to the posterior cranial fossa: sitting position, with the head firmly fixed. *Black shading:* the craniotomy site. Palpable structures include the external occipital protuberance and the mastoid

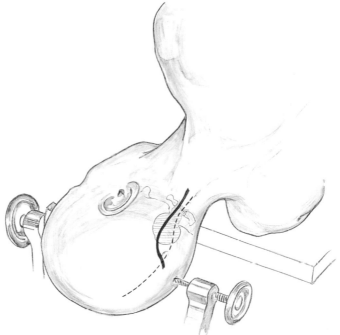

Fig. **162** Paramedian suboccipital approach to the posterior cranial fossa: lateral positioning, with firm fixing of the head. The craniotomy site and the resected atlantal arch are shown in black. The figures below represent the sitting position

Incision of Soft Tissues
(Fig. 163)

The musculature is divided as far as the occipital squama and the lateral atlantal arch. The anatomical structures are dissected free with raspatories, and explored with retractors.

Craniotomy

When the occipital squama and the dorsolateral atlantal arch have been exposed, a burr hole is made. From here, an osteoclastic enlargement to the great foramen is performed. The atlantal arch is partially resected, special attention being paid to the course of the vertebral artery. Bleeding portions of bone are treated with bone wax.

Opening the Dura
(Fig. 164)

The medially pedicled dura is opened laterally by an arcuate incision. When lifting the dura off the cerebellum, attention has to be paid to bridging veins and cortical vessels. It is not uncommon for the dura to adhere to the arachnoid.

The lateral portion of the brain stem is exposed by retraction and elevation of the cerebellar hemisphere (Fig. 165).

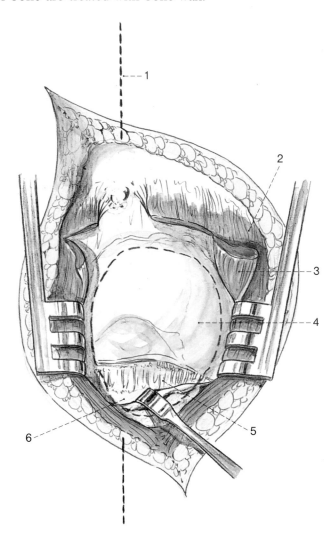

Fig. **163** The musculature has been longitudinally divided and is distracted with retractors. The periosteum is retracted. Red dashed lines mark the craniotomy area and the portion of the atlantal arch to be resected

1 Midline
2 Trapezius muscle
3 Semispinalis capitis muscle
4 Occipital bone
5 Atlanto-occipital membrane
6 Arch of the atlas

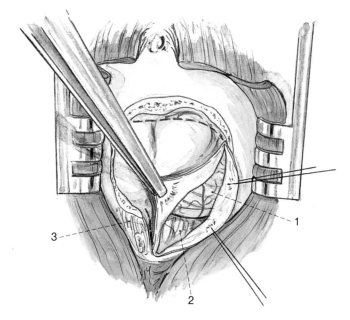

Fig. **164** After the craniotomy has been carried out and the atlantal arch has been resected, the dura is cut circumferentially, with the base directed medially. Lateral areas of the right cerebellar hemisphere and tonsil are brought into view. The dural incision can be continued along the dashed red line

1 Cerebellar hemisphere
2 Cerebellar tonsil
3 Posterior atlanto-occipital membrane

Dural and Wound Closure

The dura has to be closed in a watertight fashion. Only homologous materials should be used for replacement of dura. The musculature and the fascia are approximated, and the subcutis and cutis are sutured. Suction drains should only be used in exceptional cases.

Potential Errors and Dangers

— Hemorrhages from cut borders of the skin or the musculature during the operation
— Injuries to the cerebellar surface due to the craniotome
— Injuries to the vertebral artery during resection of the atlantal arch
— Postoperative hemorrhages from unsecured vessels of the cerebellar surface or the dura
— Cerebrospinal fluid fistula
— Soft-tissue hematoma

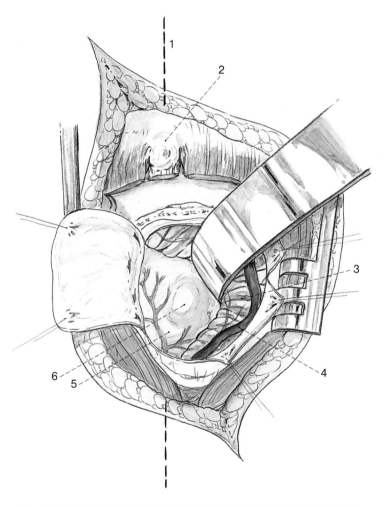

Fig. **165**   The dural flap is reflected medially and the cerebellar hemisphere has been retracted laterally-superiorly to the right, together with the posterior inferior cerebellar artery, using a soft spatula, so that the cystic brain stem tumor is visualized

1 Midline
2 External occipital protuberance
3 Cerebellar hemisphere
4 Posterior inferior cerebellar artery (PICA)
5 Medulla oblongata
6 Cystic tumor

11 Approaches to the Cervical Spine

Anterior Approach to the Cervical Spine

Typical Indications for Surgery

- Degenerative changes of the cervical spine
- Median and mediolateral prolapse of nucleus pulposus
- Replacement of vertebral body
- Injuries to cervical vertebrae
- Inflammatory bone alterations

Principal Anatomical Structures

Platysma, transverse nerve of neck, anterior jugular vein, cutaneous branch of the superior thyroid artery, superficial lamina of the cervical fascia, sternocleidomastoid muscle, sternothyroid muscle, sternohyoid muscle, omohyoid muscle, thyroid gland, internal jugular vein, superior thyroid vein, common carotid artery, superior and inferior thyroid arteries, recurrent laryngeal nerve, trachea, esophagus, long muscle of the neck (medial fibers), prevertebral lamina of the cervical fascia, cervical vertebra, intervertebral disk, anterior longitudinal ligament, spinal dura mater.

Positioning and Skin Incisions

(Fig. **166**)

The right-handed surgeon will prefer the patient's right side at the neck, because the operative field is narrowed by the mobile radiography equipment. The patient is placed in a supine position; a moderately full sandbag is put between the shoulder blades, and a suitable air cushion or a space-occupying layer of cellulose is placed below the cervical spine. In this manner the cervical spine can be sufficiently extended for the operative procedure. Owing to the underlying disease, this inclination has to be very limited; this also applies to the endotracheal intubation, regarding which the anesthetist has to be properly informed. The patient's chin remains in a median position. In the last step, the radiography equipment (C-arc) is moved into place, and its alignment toward the cervical spine is verified.

For the skin incision, longitudinal and transverse cuts can be made at various levels. If more than three cervical vertebrae are to be exposed, a skin incision at the anterior border of the sternocleidomastoid muscle is preferable. It begins below the mandible and extends to the sternum. Otherwise, use is made of a so-called half-collar incision running from the midline, in the direction of the skin fold, 7–8 cm to the

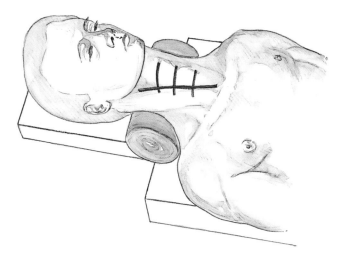

Fig. **166** Anterior approach to the cervical spine: positioning and incisions. There are pads under the neck and between the shoulder-blades. The head is inclined only slightly. The longitudinal incision at the border of the sternocleidomastoid muscle serves to expose several vertebrae; the half-collar incisions can be used for the approach to 2–3 cervical vertebrae

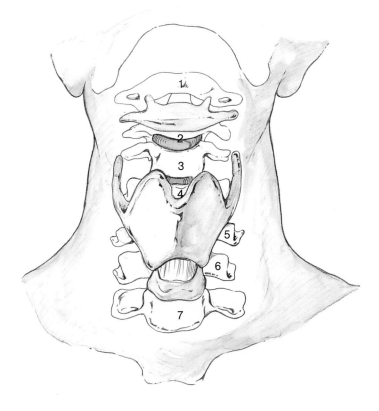

Fig. **167** Orientation points for choice of the optimal level of the half-collar incision

side and generally slightly past the anterior border of the sternocleidomastoid muscle. Choosing the optimal level relative to the targeted cervical vertebra is important for the placement of these transverse incisions (Fig. **167**). For the C2–C3 vertebrae, this is the hyoid bone; for C4–C5, it is the thyroid cartilage; for C5–C6, the cricoid cartilage, and for C7–T1, 3 cm above the clavicle.

Dissection of the Superficial Layers
(Fig. **168**)

After transection of the platysma the superficial vessels and small cutaneous nerves are usually readily identified. Some of these structures can therefore be retracted. A smaller proportion of them are coagulated, ligated, and divided.

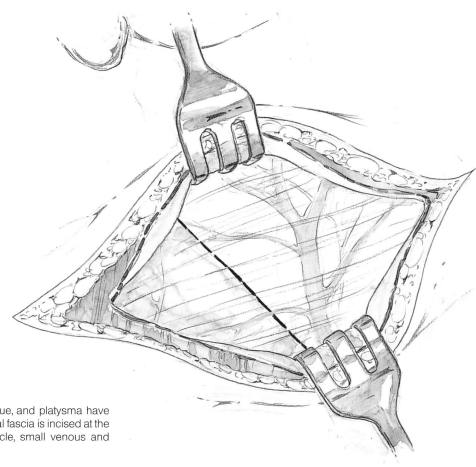

Fig. **168** The skin, subcutaneous adipose tissue, and platysma have been divided. The superficial lamina of the cervical fascia is incised at the medial border of the sternocleidomastoid muscle, small venous and nerve branches being transected

Dissection in the Plane of Muscles and Soft Tissues
(Fig. **169**)

With the aid of a longitudinal incision, exploration in the depth is carried out using both sharp and blunt dissection alongside the anterior border of the sternocleidomastoid muscle and lateral to the subhyoid musculature. The superior venter of the omohyoid muscle is divided, and the median layer of the cervical fascia is opened. Several obliquely coursing veins from the thyroid area are in part coagulated and in part ligated. Individual slender nerves from the deep ansa cervicalis have to be divided, and cannot be retracted from the approach site.

The ensuing procedure is best performed with both index fingers. The carotid artery, the internal jugular vein, the vagus nerve and, medially, the trachea, the thyroid, and the muscles can be palpated and separated from one another. The esophageal walls, which have low resistance, can be protected from injury in this fashion. The same purpose is served by insertion of a stomach tube. At this point, the finger is able to palpate the special shape of the immediately subjacent vertebrae; the finger can also detect radiographically revealed deformities (V-shaped degenerative changes of endplates or fractures) (Fig. **170**).

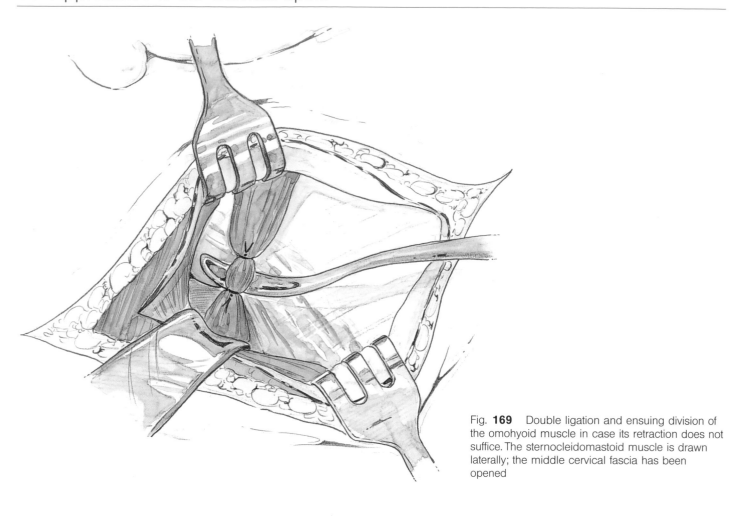

Fig. **169**   Double ligation and ensuing division of the omohyoid muscle in case its retraction does not suffice. The sternocleidomastoid muscle is drawn laterally; the middle cervical fascia has been opened

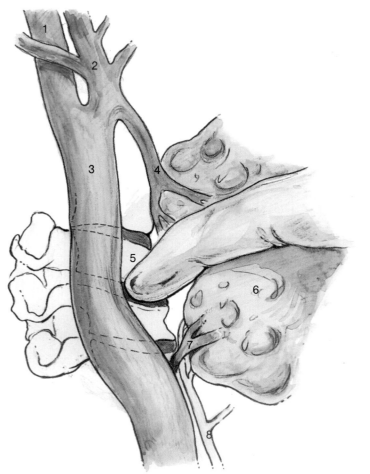

Fig. **170**   The palpating and dissecting finger as it reaches the usually deformed endplate of a degeneratively altered cervical vertebra. The thyroid and the esophagus have been retracted medially and the common carotid artery laterally. At the superior pole of the thyroid, the superior thyroid artery can be palpated, and at the inferior pole the inferior thyroid artery and the inferior laryngeal (recurrent) nerve can be palpated

1   Internal carotid artery
2   External carotid artery
3   Common carotid artery
4   Superior thyroid artery
5   Cervical vertebra
6   Thyroid gland
7   Inferior thyroid artery
8   Recurrent laryngeal nerve

Among the anatomical structures, the recurrent laryngeal nerve and the thyroid vessels require special attention. In a high approach, this also applies to branches of the superficial ansa cervicalis. The superior thyroid artery arising from the external carotid artery, as well as the lingual and facial arteries, can be ligated if absolutely necessary. In most cases, however, they can be bluntly retracted superiorly. The anatomical site is shown in Figure **171.** The site for operation on the lowest cervical vertebrae is crossed by the infe-

rior thyroid artery, which generally has to be divided between ligatures. In this area, the sympathetic trunk with its stellate ganglion may also come into view. Laterally, it is accompanied by the vertebral artery shortly after its origin from the subclavian artery. Consequently, the cervical pleura, too, is in the immediate proximity and exposed to injury. On the left side, finally, the thoracic duct has to be identified and spared (Fig. **172**).

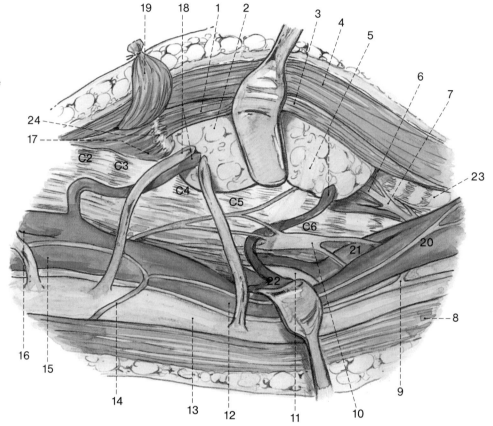

Fig. **171** Topographic anatomy of the middle region of the cervical spine as viewed by the surgeon

1 Thyrohyoid muscle
2 Thyroid
3 Sternothyroid muscle
4 Sternohyoid muscle
5 Inferior thyroid artery and vein
6 Inferior laryngeal (recurrent) nerve
7 Esophagus
8 Sternocleidomastoid muscle
9 Vagus nerve
10 Sympathetic trunk and stellate ganglion
11 Vertebral vein
12 Common carotid artery
13 Internal jugular vein
14 Deep ansa cervicalis (inferior root)
15 External carotid artery
16 Internal carotid artery
17 Pharynx
18 Superior thyroid artery and vein
19 Omohyoid muscle (divided)
20 Brachiocephalic trunk
21 Subclavian artery
22 Thyrocervical trunk
23 Trachea
24 Thyroid cartilage
25 Middle thyroid vein

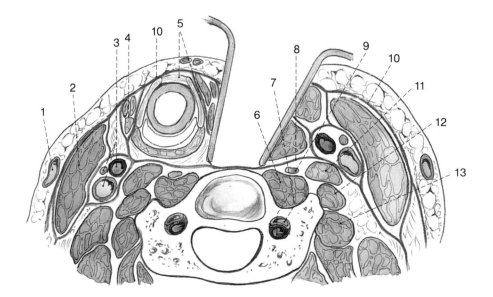

Fig. **172** Anatomical cross-section between the second and third cervical vertebrae, with intubation tube inserted and retractor applied

1 External jugular vein
2 Sternocleidomastoid muscle
3 Common carotid artery, internal jugular vein, and vagus nerve
4 Infrahyoid muscle
5 Pretracheal lamina of the cervical fascia
6 Long muscle of the neck
7 Vertebral artery and vein
8 Prevertebral lamina of the cervical fascia
9 Sympathetic trunk
10 Superficial lamina of the cervical fascia
11 Long muscle of the head
12 Anterior scalene muscle
13 Middle scalene muscle

Dissection in the Area of the Deep Cervical Fascia
(Fig. 173)

The deep layer of the cervical fascia can now be divided in the midline and retracted to the sides. Ensuing bipolar and monopolar coagulation of the insertions of the longus colli muscle in its pars recta is important in order to prevent troublesome oozing hemorrhages from this area. A rubber-insulated slender probe is needed for monopolar coagulation.

After this, the two muscle parts can be bluntly retracted to the side and kept in this position with the aid of special spreaders of different lengths. Still overlying the spine are the anterior longitudinal ligament and the vertebral periosteum, which are likewise retracted. In this phase, the desired level of the operation has to be finally determined with the aid of the mobile radiography equipment and documented by a concluding radiograph. The subsequent operation on the spinal column then follows.

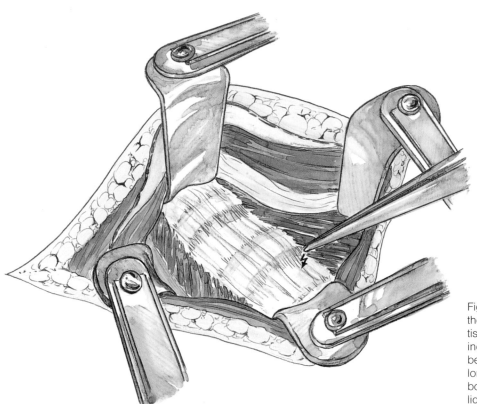

Fig. **173**   Special spreaders have been applied; they keep the adjacent muscles, vessels, and soft tissues out of the operative field. At least in elderly individuals, the common carotid artery should not be retracted. The easily bleeding insertions of the long muscle of the neck lateral to the vertebral bodies are coagulated. The anterior longitudinal ligament and the periosteum can be opened

Wound Closure

Soft-tissue sutures are hardly necessary when short transverse incisions have been used; after a longitudinal incision, approximation of the musculature is required, and the divided portions of the omohyoid muscle are rejoined. Whether a drain should be used depends on the extent of the local bleeding tendency; it is therefore rarely needed.

Potential Errors and Dangers

— Appreciable inclination of the head should be avoided during intubation and positioning
— Injury to the esophagus, common carotid artery, vagus nerve, recurrent laryngeal nerve and thyroid vessels by instruments
— Injury to the cervical pleura, sympathetic trunk, vertebral artery, or vertebral nerve during deep dissection
— Omission of preventive coagulation at the insertions of the longus colli muscle at the vertebrae
— Deviation from the midline

Mediolateral Approach to the Cervical Spine

Typical Indications for Surgery

- Degenerative changes of the cervical spine
- Mediolateral and lateral prolapse of nucleus pulposus
- Exposure of vertebral artery in case of constriction by uncarthrosis
- Special types of injuries to cervical vertebrae
- Inflammatory changes of the bone and adjacent soft tissues

Principal Anatomical Structures

Platysma, cervical fascia (superficial and pretracheal laminae), anterior jugular vein, transverse nerve of the neck, sternohyoid and sternothyroid muscles, omohyoid muscle, trachea and larynx, thyroid, esophagus, sternocleidomastoid muscle, common carotid artery, internal and external carotid artery, internal and external jugular veins, vagus nerve, sympathetic trunk, phrenic nerve, superior and inferior thyroid artery and vein, cervical fascia (prevertebral lamina), longus colli muscle, anterior and middle scalene muscles, cervical vertebra with transverse processes, intertransverse muscles, carotid tubercle, longus capitis muscle, vertebral artery and veins, spinal root, cervical pleura.

Positioning and Skin Incision

(Fig. 174)

The patient is placed in a supine position; a well-fitting sandbag or a space-occupying layer of cellulose is put under the neck. Extension of the cervical spine has to be kept

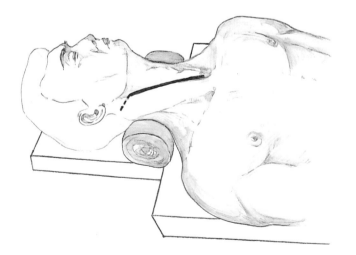

Fig. **174** Anterior approach to the lateral cervical spine for an uncoforaminotomy: positioning and incision

within narrow limits, in view of the underlying disease. This also has to be borne in mind with the endotracheal intubation, about which the anesthetist therefore has to be properly warned. The patient's head is turned slightly to the opposite side.

Next, the mobile radiography equipment (C-arc) is set up so that films can be obtained intraoperatively. The side of the skin incision depends on the underlying process.

The cosmetically preferable collar incision cannot be expanded upward or downward. The incision is therefore made alongside the medial border of the sternocleidomastoid muscle. Extension of the incision into the mandibular angle is directed upward toward the sternocleidomastoid muscle.

Dissection of the Superficial Layer
(Fig. **175**)

When the more or less fully developed platysma has also been divided in the direction of the skin incision, the superficial layer of the cervical fascia is reached, and this is similarly divided. In this step, individual small veins as well as small cutaneous nerves have to be transected if they cannot be retracted from the operative field.

Dissection in the Vascular Layer
(Fig. **176**)

Since it is generally the cervical vertebrae C5–C6 that are targeted, dissection and division of the omohyoid muscle is unavoidable in most cases. It is first ligated, both to prevent hemorrhages and for the purpose of displacing and rejoining the stumps.

Retraction of the thyroid to the contralateral side often necessitates ligation and division of the superior and, less commonly, the inferior thyroid arteries and veins. In these cases, very close attention has to be paid – particularly on the right side of the neck – to the recurrent laryngeal nerve, so that the blunt or sharp dissection has to be carried out under optimal illumination, and possibly with the aid of optical magnification. The operative field encompasses the sympathetic trunk with the stellate ganglion and the vertebral nerve. The latter can be divided. At the end of this phase of the dissection, the thyroid and the esophagus are retracted medially, and the vessels laterally. The retractor should not be used on the vessels; they should be removed to the side with a suitable narrow instrument (dissecting swab, slender elevator, narrow and soft spatula).

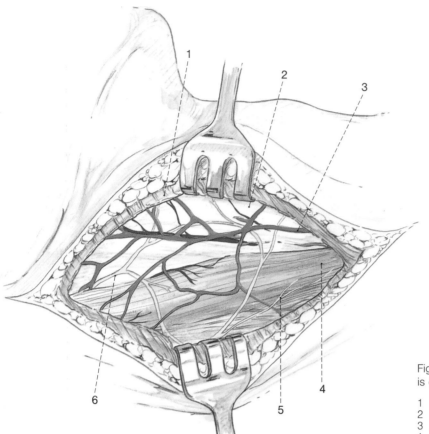

Fig. **175** Dissection of the superficial layers. The fascia is opened at the border of the sternocleidomastoid muscle

1 Platysma
2 Cervical fascia (superficial lamina)
3 Anterior jugular vein
4 Sternocleidomastoid muscle
5 Transverse nerve of the neck (inferior branch)
6 Cervical branch of the facial nerve

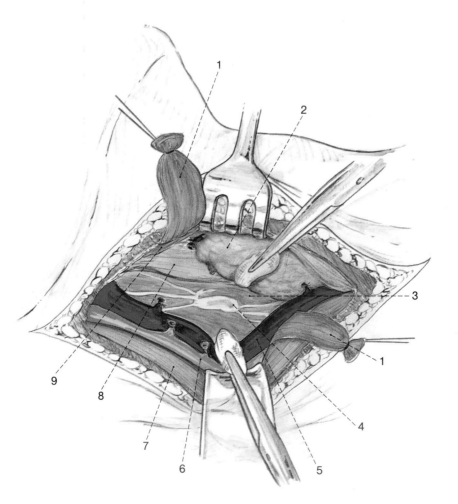

Fig. **176** Dissection of the vascular layer. The omohyoid muscle has been divided; the thyroid has been retracted medially and the neurovascular bundle laterally. This exposes the long muscle of the neck and the sympathetic trunk

1 Omohyoid muscle
2 Thyroid
3 Long muscle of neck
4 Sympathetic trunk with ganglion
5 Common carotid artery
6 Internal jugular vein
7 Sternocleidomastoid muscle
8 Cervical fascia (pretracheal lamina)
9 Sternothyroid muscle

Dissection in the Muscular Layer
(Fig. **177**)

In the next step, the longitudinal portion of the longus colli muscle can be retracted medially; for this purpose, slender raspatories are required in the areas of vertebral bodies and transverse processes. The readily palpable carotid tubercle of the sixth cervical vertebra and the overlying anterior transverse tubercle of the fifth cervical vertebra are exposed after detachment of the local insertions of the corresponding parts of the longus colli and capitis muscles. This may bring into view the vertebral artery and its accom-

panying veins, which completely cover it in many cases. The goal of this phase of the operation is exposure of the anterior transverse tubercles of the transverse processes, as well as of the transverse processes themselves. This makes it possible to develop exposure of the vertebral artery, which generally enters from below in the area of the transverse process of the sixth cervical vertebra, and also expose its further course in the contiguous intervertebral foramina.

The anatomical relations are shown, with particular reference to the deep location of the vertebral artery, in Figure **178**.

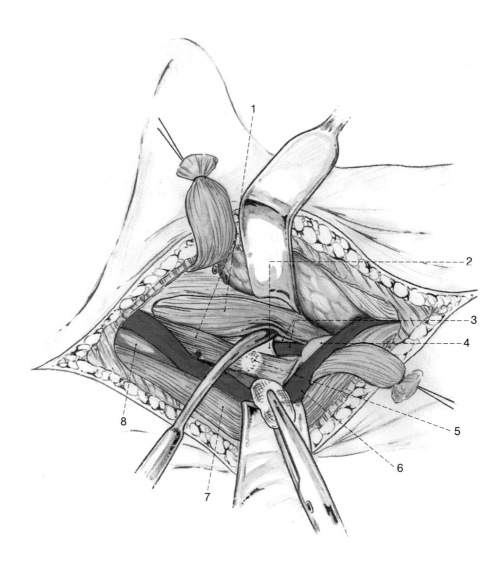

Fig. **177** Dissection of muscle layer. The thyroid and the vessels have been displaced; the long muscle of neck can be transposed medially; its insertions at the carotid tubercle are transected. This brings the vertebral artery and accompanying veins into view

1 Long muscle of neck
2 Transverse process of the sixth cervical vertebra
3 Vertebral vein and artery
4 Sympathetic trunk
5 Carotid tubercle
6 Common carotid artery
7 Sternocleidomastoid muscle
8 Internal jugular vein

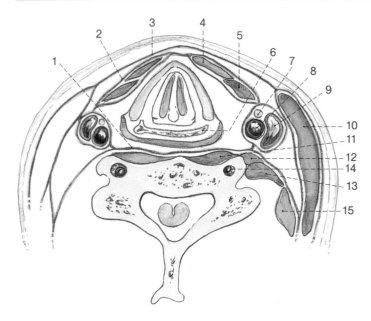

Fig. **178**   Cross-section through the neck at the level of the fifth cervical vertebra. The fasciae are highlighted

 1   Cervical fascia (prevertebral lamina)
 2   Cervical fascia (pretracheal lamina)
 3   Cervical fascia (superficial lamina)
 4   Sternohyoid muscle
 5   Sternothyroid muscle
 6   Laryngopharynx
 7   Vagus nerve
 8   Common carotid artery
 9   Internal jugular vein
10   Sternocleidomastoid muscle
11   Long muscle of the neck
12   Long muscle of the head
13   Anterior scalene muscle
14   Vertebral artery and vein
15   Middle scalene muscle

Wound Closure

After meticulous hemostasis, the platysma, if sufficiently thick, is sutured over a suction drain. The skin and subcutaneous adipose tissue are closed with interrupted sutures. The fascial layers require no special closure.

Potential Errors and Dangers

— Excessive inclination of the head during intubation and positioning
— Injury to the esophagus, common carotid artery, vagus and recurrent laryngeal nerves, and to thyroid vessels, due to instruments
— Injury to the cervical pleura, sympathetic trunk, and vertebral artery during deep dissection
— Injury to the vertebral artery
— Insufficient hemostasis of vertebral veins
— Alteration of the brachial plexus due to excessive traction from retractors

Posterior Approach to the Cervical Spine

Typical Indications for Surgery

— Extraspinal and intraspinal neoplasms
— Degenerative changes
— Dilatations of the vertebral canal

Principal Anatomical Structures

Splenius capitis muscle, semispinalis capitis muscle, minor and major rectus capitis posterior muscles, inferior oblique muscle of the head, semispinalis cervicis muscle, rhomboid muscle, posterior inferior serratus muscle, trapezius muscle, spinalis muscle, interspinal muscle, multifidus muscle, nuchal ligament, interspinal ligament, spinous process, spinous arch, spinal dura mater, azygos vein of the neck, azygos vein of the back, deep cervical artery and vein, posterior internal vertebral venous plexus, vertebral artery and vein, intervertebral veins, spinal medulla, cervical nerve, spinal ganglion, ventral and dorsal roots of the cervical nerve, denticulate ligament.

Positioning and Skin Incision

(Fig. **179**)

The patient is placed in the sitting position, with the head bent slightly forward. The legs are slightly raised. The head is firmly fixed.

The skin incision should not be exactly in the midline, so that wound healing may not be adversely affected by reduced blood flow through this midline. Accordingly, the incision is made in a slightly arcuate fashion. Larger incisions are somewhat S-shaped.

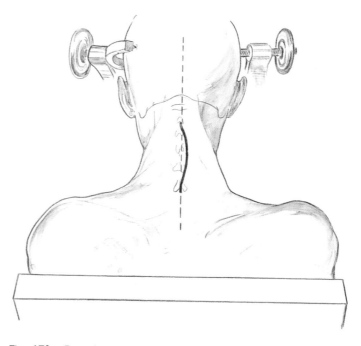

Fig. **179** Posterior approach to the cervical spine: positioning and incision. The spinous processes of cervical vertebrae 1 – 5 are marked, as is the posterior basicranial border

Dissection of Musculature

(Fig. 180)

When the fascia has been longitudinally incised, the tendinous portion between the bilateral muscles can be developed. Depending on the level of the segment in which the operation is performed, the investing muscle layers vary in number and thickness. In most cases, dissection in the depth is performed in layers immediately alongside the spinous processes and the interspinal ligaments connecting them, using cutting diathermy. The retractor is moved each time to the next, deeper layer; small hemorrhages are stopped at once. The resulting trenches can be packed with saline-impregnated gauze in order to arrest residual minor hemorrhages. Finally, the attachments of the vertebral arches to their spinous processes, lined by the intervertebral ligaments, are exposed.

An overview of the major muscles involved that are encountered upon posterior exposure of the cervical region is shown in Figure 181.

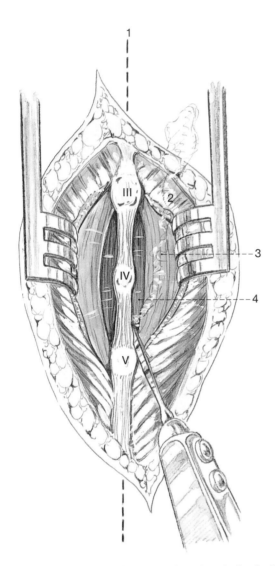

Fig. **180** The skin and adipose tissue have been longitudinally divided. The underlying muscle layers are separated in layers, close to the bone

1 Midline
2 Splenius capitis muscle
3 Semispinalis capitis muscle
4 Semispinalis cervicis muscle
III, IV, V Spinous processes of the corresponding cervical vertebrae

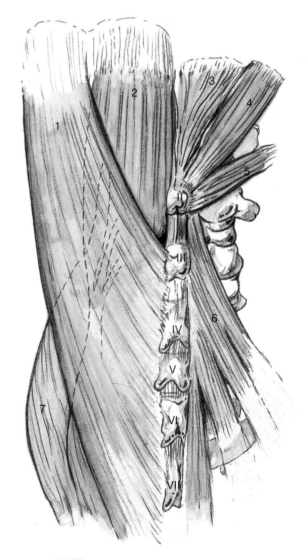

Fig. **181** Muscles in the dorsal region of the cervical spine

1 Splenius capitis muscle
2 Semispinalis capitis muscle
3 Rectus capitis posterior minor muscle
4 Rectus capitis posterior major muscle
5 Inferior oblique muscle of the head
6 Semispinalis cervicis muscle
7 Splenius cervicis muscle
I–VII Spinous processes of the corresponding cervical vertebrae

Laminectomy at the Level of the Fourth and Fifth Cervical Vertebrae
(Fig. 182)

The entire musculature, which has been divided in the midline, can finally be distracted with a suitable spreader. The spinous process or processes are usually ablated at their base with a Luer bone forceps. Punches or water-cooled burrs prove satisfactory for resection of the adjoining portions of the lamina. The lateral procedure is determined by the extent of the targeted process. However, an effort is made not to injure the vertebral joints.

If the underlying process permits, a hemilaminectomy can be performed, in which additional intraspinal space is gained by obliquely drilling off the medial portions of the spinous process base.

Opening the Dura
(Fig. 183)

If the targeted process is situated extradurally, or if a decompressive operation is planned, the dura is not opened.

In other cases, it is lifted with a pointed needle and incised longitudinally after retraction of the investing fatty tissue. Several elevation sutures keep the operative field open and stop small epidural hemorrhages. Inspection of the operative site, identification of accompanying and supply vessels, and planning of the operation on the pathological process are generally performed with the aid of optical magnification.

An overview of the anatomical structures involved is given in Figure 184. Special mention should be made of hemi-

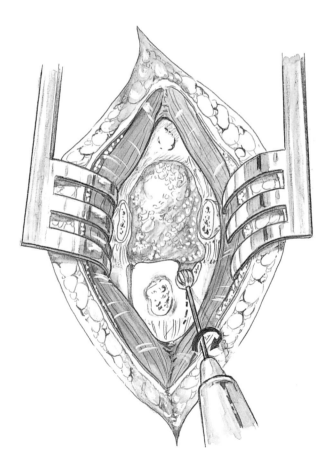

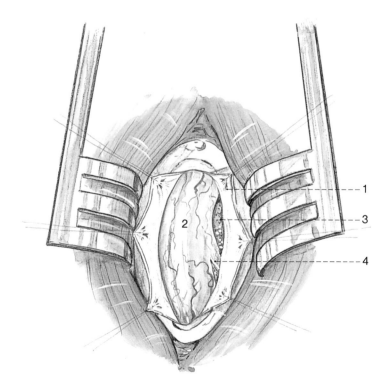

Fig. **182** The musculature is distracted with a retractor. Using fine punches or a microdrill, the vertebral arches, including their spinous processes, are mobilized and ablated. The epidural fatty tissue comes into view

Fig. **183** Following retraction of the epidural fatty tissue, the dura can bc longitudinally incised and retracted laterally with retention sutures. The intradural extramedullary tumor located ventrolaterally on the right side is now visualized

1 Dura mater
2 Spinal cord
3 Tumor
4 Spinal root

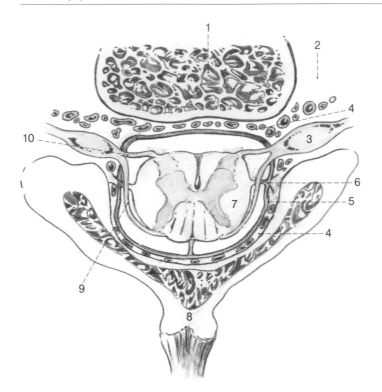

laminectomy for exposure of lateral nucleus pulposus prolapses; this is shown in Figures **185** and **186**. Following separation of the musculature with the cutting diathermy, the periosteum is retracted laterally; the two muscles are held apart with a retractor. A kidney-shaped opening is drilled into the vertebral arches; burrs or punches are then used to extend the opening as far as the vertebral articulation, the lateral joint surfaces being preserved. Bleeding portions of the epidural venous plexus should be controlled using bipolar coagulation. Now the nerve root can be dissected free. In some cases, the posterior longitudinal ligament has to be incised in order to reach the subligamentous space.

Fig. **184**   Cross-section through the middle cervical spine

 1 Cervical vertebra
 2 Vertebral artery
 3 Spinal ganglion
 4 Anterior and posterior internal vertebral plexus
 5 Spinal dura mater
 6 Denticulate ligament
 7 Spinal cord
 8 Spinous process
 9 Dorsal root
10 Ventral root

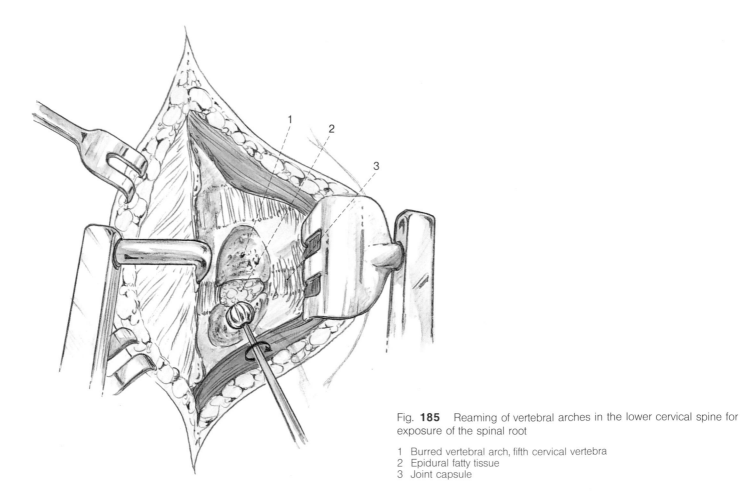

Fig. **185**   Reaming of vertebral arches in the lower cervical spine for exposure of the spinal root

1 Burred vertebral arch, fifth cervical vertebra
2 Epidural fatty tissue
3 Joint capsule

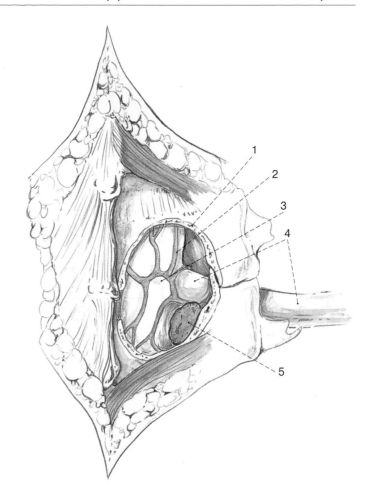

Fig. **186**   Exposure of a nucleus pulposus prolapse under the axilla of the spinal root (lateral portions are indicated transparently)

1 Cut border of the arch of the fifth cervical vertebra
2 Epidural venous plexus
3 Dura-invested cervical medulla
4 Spinal root
5 Nucleus pulposus prolapse

Wound Closure

The dura can be closed with interrupted or continuous sutures. This is followed by careful inspection of hemostasis in the epidural space.

The musculature should be sutured in as many layers as possible to minimize impairment of the gliding function among the muscles and to allow rapid wound healing.

Skin sutures can be tied individually as a rule, but they may also be placed continuously.

Potential Errors and Dangers

— Inadequate support of the head before the operation
— Injury to larger paravertebral vessels due to deviation from the midline
— Injuries to intradural structures due to lack of protection against bone burrs used in laminectomy
— Substantial postoperative blood loss due to inadequate closure of vessels during the operation
— Air embolism

Transsoral Approach to the Two Uppermost Cervical Vertebrae

Selected Indications for Surgery

— Ventral spinal tumors at this segment level
— Posttraumatic states, e.g., fractures of the dens
— Inflammatory conditions, e.g., epidural empyemas

Principal Anatomical Structures

Palatopharyngeal arch, palatoglossal arch, soft palate, palatine uvula, palatine tonsil, superior constrictor muscle of the pharynx, long muscle of the head, long muscle of the neck, anterior atlanto-occipital membrane, anterior tubercle of the atlas, body of the axis, vertebral artery.

Positioning and Incision

(Fig. **187**)

The indication for preoperative tracheotomy is discussed with the anesthetist; the probability of postoperative respiratory depression will make a decision in favor of tracheotomy more likely. An experienced anesthetist will know how to pass the tube far laterally so as to avoid any added interference in the medial operative field.

The obviously heightened risk of infection associated with this approach necessitates the use of antibiotic cover both before and after the operation. Disinfection of the pharyngeal wall has a certain reassuring effect.

The patient's head is extended backward and downward; its restraint by a firm headrest, which is fitted directly into the head of the operating table, has been found advisable. Use of a special gag which keeps the tongue out of the operative field by a plate is essential. The uvula and the soft palate have to be displaced cranially by means of a slender blunt hook or a strong suture.

Exploration of the Posterior Pharyngeal Wall

(Fig. **188**)

Using optical magnification, the posterior wall of the pharynx is readily visualized, so that the location of the longitudinal incision can be selected.

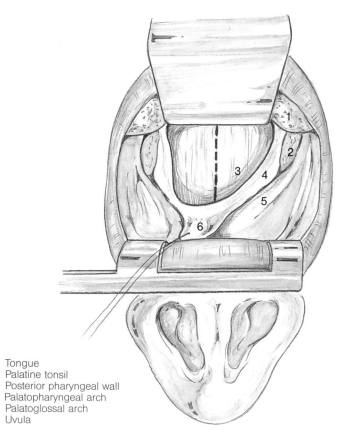

1   Tongue
2   Palatine tonsil
3   Posterior pharyngeal wall
4   Palatopharyngeal arch
5   Palatoglossal arch
6   Uvula

Fig. **187**   Transoral approach to the cervical spine: positioning and incision

Fig. **188**   Visualization of the pharynx, retraction of the uvula, and marking of the mucosa-soft tissue incision (red dashed line)

Division of the Posterior Pharyngeal Wall
(Fig. 189)

Following the mucosa, the superior constrictor muscle of the pharynx is likewise incised longitudinally and distracted. The readily palpable anterior tubercle of the atlas and the anterior wall of the second cervical vertebra may serve as guides.

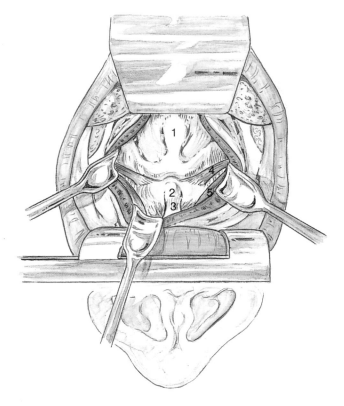

Fig. **190**   The soft tissues have been retracted, so that the first and second cervical vertebrae can be developed

1 Body of axis
2 Anterior tubercle of atlas
3 Anterior atlanto-occipital membrane
4 Long muscle of neck
5 Long muscle of head

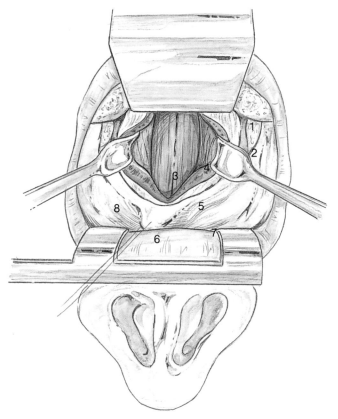

Fig. **189**   The posterior wall of the pharynx is split in layers

1 Tongue
2 Palatine tonsil
3 Long muscle of the neck
4 Long muscle of the head
5 Superior constrictor muscle of the pharynx
6 Uvula
7 Soft palate
8 Palatopharyngeal arch

Exploration of the Anterior Sides of the Two Upper Cervical Vertebrae
(Fig. 190)

When the underlying longus colli muscle has been split longitudinally, the transected layers can be dissected toward the sides with slender raspatories to bring the two upper cervical vertebrae into view. None of the dissections, however, should exceed a width of 2–2.5 cm, so that the vertebral artery is not compromised. On the epistropheus in particular, lateral dissection should be more limited.

These anatomical relations are once more brought into focus in Figure **191**.

The exposed operative field can be well developed and prepared for the ensuing operative steps with the aid of slender elastic spatulas.

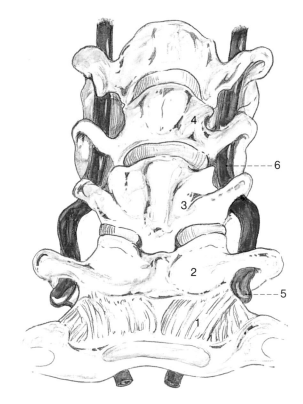

Fig. **191**   The course of the vertebral artery in the area of the upper and middle cervical spine

1 Anterior atlanto-occipital membrane
2 Atlas
3 Epistropheus
4 Third cervical vertebra
5 Vertebral artery (transverse part)
6 Vertebral artery (vertebral part)

Wound Closure

The two transected muscle layers (long muscle of the neck, superior constrictor muscle of the pharynx) are closed with interrupted sutures; an attempt may be made to suture the mucosa.

Potential Errors and Dangers

— Unstable positioning
— Deviation from the midline
— Excessively lateral dissection on the anterior vertebral surfaces
— Injuries to the vertebral artery
— Injuries to the glossopharyngeal and hypoglossal nerves in the retromandibular fossa
— Injuries to the anterior spinal artery

12 Approaches to the Thoracic Spine

Posterior Approach to the Thoracic Spine

Typical Indications for Surgery

- Tumors
- Vascular malformations
- Posttraumatic states
- Bone compression

Principal Anatomical Structures

Trapezius muscle, greater and lesser rhomboid muscles, latissimus dorsi muscle, longissimus muscles of the neck and thorax, posterior inferior serratus muscle, thoracolumbar fascia, supraspinal ligament, spinalis thoracis muscle, anterior and posterior longitudinal ligaments, posterior intercostal arteries and veins, vertebral venous plexus, spinous processes, vertebral arch, vertebral body, intercostal nerves, spinal medulla, spinal nerve, ventral root, dorsal root, denticulate ligament, spinal ganglion, spinal dura mater, ribs, pleura.

Positioning and Incision
(Figs. 192 and 193)

The patient may be in a lateral or a prone position; the choice is determined in large part by the patient's condition, the anesthetist's views, and a possible further spread of the tumor to surrounding areas – but also by the surgeon's own personal preferences.

To guard against reduced blood flow, the skin incision should not be made exactly in the midline; instead, a mildly arcuate or S-shaped incision may be performed.

Incision of the Top Muscle Layer
(Fig. 194)

Using cutting diathermy in most cases, the tendinous fibers of the top muscle layer (trapezius, rhomboid muscles) are divided directly at the spinous processes, and the hemorrhages are controlled, followed by application of retractors.

Retraction of the Musculature
(Fig. 195)

The musculature can be detached subperiosteally and retracted laterally with raspatories and elevators. The resulting gap is packed with hot saline-impregnated gauze so that more diffuse hemorrhages can be stopped without delay. Visibly bleeding vessels may be closed bipolarly.

The anatomical relations are shown in Figures 196 and 197.

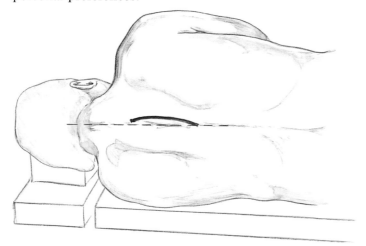

Fig. **192**   Posterior approach to the thoracic spine: lateral positioning and incision. Palpable fixation points comprise the prominent vertebra, other spinous processes and, occasionally, the last rib. These points are not sufficient for an exact localization of the level

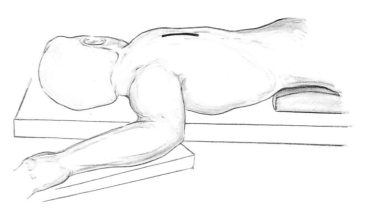

Fig. **193**   Posterior approach to the thoracic spine: prone positioning and incision. The remarks under Figure **192** also apply to the palpable fixation points here

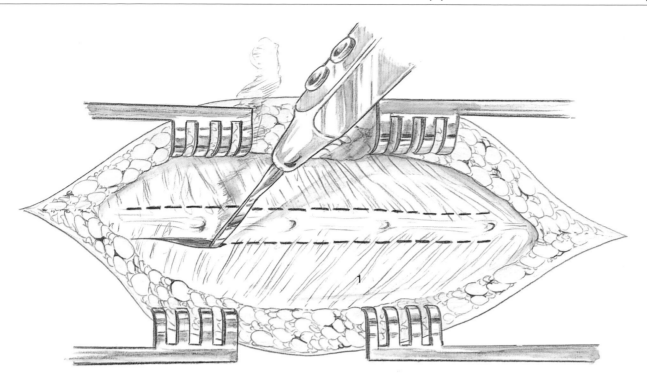

Fig. **194**   The incised skin and subcutaneous adipose tissue are distracted with retractors. Closely alongside the palpable and visible spinous processes, the fascia is bilaterally incised and then the musculature (dashed red line); the cutting diathermy is particularly suitable for this purpose. Marking of the level must be performed radiologically prior to the operation

1   Trapezius muscle and thoracolumbar fascia

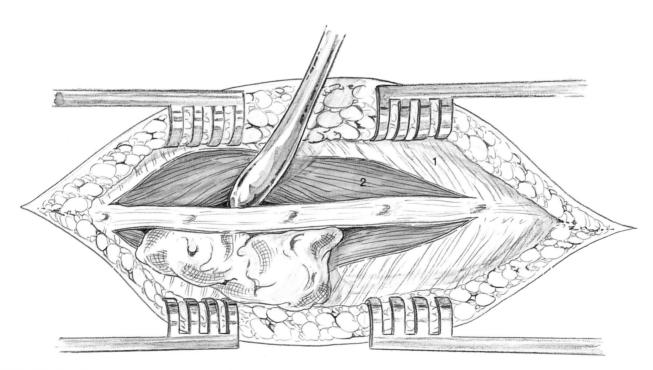

Fig. **195**   With the aid of elevators, the musculature is retracted subperiosteally as far as the base of the spinous processes. Gauze strips impregnated with hot saline solution are introduced into the resulting cavity; this contributes substantially to hemostasis

1   Trapezius muscle and thoracolumbar fascia
2   Erector muscle of the spine

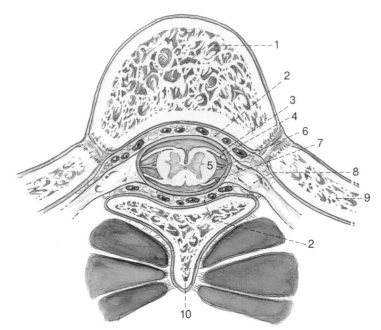

Fig. **196**   Cross-section through the fifth thoracic vertebra, as seen from below

1   Fifth thoracic vertebra
2   Anterior and posterior internal vertebral plexus
3   Spinal dura mater
4   Radix anterior
5   Spinal cord
6   Denticulate ligament
7   Radix posterior
8   Spinal ganglion
9   Fifth rib
10 Spinous process

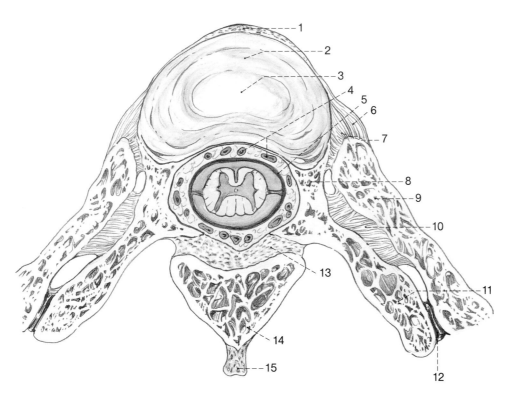

Fig. **197**   Cross-section at the level of the intervertebral disk between the second and third thoracic vertebrae (viewed from above)

1   Anterior longitudinal ligament
2   Annulus fibrosus
3   Nucleus pulposus
4   Epidural fatty tissue with anterior and posterior internal vertebral venous plexus
5   Spinal dura mater
6   Radiate ligament of the head of the rib
7   Interarticular ligament of the head of the rib
8   Pedicle of the vertebral arch
9   Head of the rib
10 Costotransverse ligament
11 Transverse process of the third thoracic vertebra
12 Costotransverse articulation
13 Ligamentum flavum
14 Spinous process of the second thoracic vertebra
15 Supraspinal ligament

Removal of the Vertebral Arches
(Fig. **198**)

Following retraction of the periosteum (inset on the left), the vertebral arches to be removed can be resected with punches (inset on the right) or cooled burrs. By milling off the base of the spinous process, this hemilaminectomy can be markedly enlarged, thus commensurately widening the field of vision without further reducing the stability of the vertebral column in the approach to an intraspinal process. Hemorrhages from the epidural space will be arrested after cautious bipolar coagulation or application of cellulose hemostatic netting (Surgicel).

Removal of the Spinous Processes
(Fig. **199**)

If a laminectomy has been planned from the start, the osseous part of the operation begins with removal of the selected spinous process or processes with a strong sharp bone instrument, such as a Liston or Luer rongeur, for example. A remnant of the process base always remains so that the strongest portion of the bone is left in place. The uppermost and lowermost interspinal ligaments in the area of the laminectomy are transected.

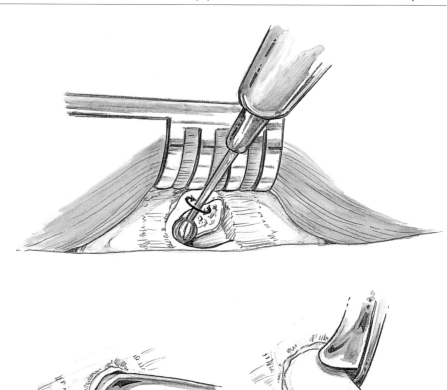

Fig. **198** For a hemilaminectomy, the spinous process is left in place. At its base, the vertebral arch is freed of periosteum (inset below left) and thereafter removed with punches (inset, below right) or a burr head

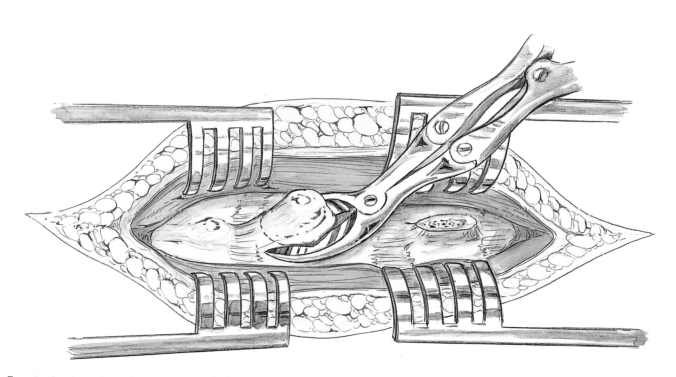

Fig. **199** For a laminectomy, the spinous processes in the area to be exposed are removed first

Opening the Vertebral Canal
(Fig. 200)

The actual wall of the bony spinal canal is opened with slender punches or with cooled burrs. The epidural fatty tissue is visualized; not uncommonly, it is permeated by several veins, which are carefully secured by bipolar coagulation.

Laminotomy
(Fig. 201)

In neurosurgery, this is understood to mean an en-bloc resection of vertebral arches and spinous processes with a view to final reimplantation of the complete bone-ligament preparation. The procedure is used preferentially in growing patients; whether the preparation will grow concomitantly cannot be safely predicted, however.

Dissection is performed with slender cutting instruments (oscillating saw, Gigli saw, strong scalpel, laser beam) either in both of the bordering intervertebral spaces, or transversely through the bone to the posterior longitudinal ligament. This is followed by an analogous division in the region of the arch and between the arches, so that the complete preparation can be carefully stripped from the underlying layers and packed off in a moist state during the following operation. At the end of the operation, the specimen is reinserted at its site of removal with the aid of retention sutures.

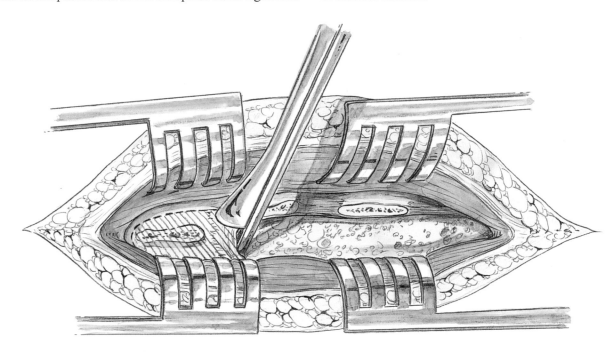

Fig. **200**   This is followed by removal of the bases of the ablated spinous processes and of the adjoining arch components (red shaded areas) and the connecting ligament sections. Both punches and burrs can be used for this purpose. Finally, the epidural fatty tissue, below which a more or less strongly developed venous plexus is found, lies exposed

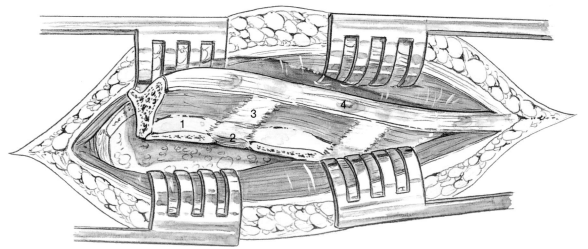

1 Vertebral arch (divided)
2 Flaval ligaments
3 Interspinal ligaments
4 Spinous process and
   supraspinal ligament

Fig. **201**   In the special form of laminotomy involving en-bloc removal of the investing parts of bone, the undermined vertebral arches and the upper and lower confining interspaces between the spinous processes have been divided so that the entire preparation can be taken out and reinserted at the end of the operation

Opening the Dura

(Fig. 202)

After being lifted with a fine point, the dura can be longitudinally incised with a knife or scissors. Elevation sutures provide for optimal utilization of the approach.

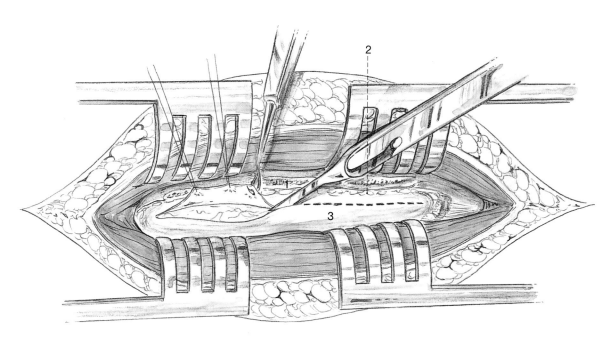

Fig. **202** The adipose tissue has been retracted, and bleeding veins from the plexus have undergone bipolar coagulation. The exposed dura (red dashed line) can be opened by a longitudinal incision and then elevated by suture. The spinal cord and pathological processes are now visualized

1 Vertebral arch (divided)
2 Retracted epidural fatty tissue
3 Spinal dura mater with incision line

Wound Closure

The dura is closed with interrupted or continuous sutures; in the latter method, knots should be tied intermittently to avoid subjecting the suture to longitudinal tension.

The musculature is closed with interrupted sutures in several layers. Continuous sutures should be avoided, so that the muscle layers are not unduly hindered in gliding past one another. Whether or not a suction drain is inserted will depend on the individual findings.

Skin sutures may again be either interrupted or continuous.

Potential Errors and Dangers

— Overlooked blood loss during the operation from the soft-tissue area; this is particularly dangerous in children
— Missing the targeted vertebral level owing to inadequate marking procedures
— Injury to the spinal medulla
— Insufficient control of hemorrhages from the spinal venous plexus
— Inadequate closure of the dura

Dorsolateral Approach to the Thoracic Spine (Costotransversectomy)

Typical Indications for Surgery

— Inflammatory foci in the thoracic spine
— Tumorous processes in the thoracic spine
— Intervertebral disk prolapses in the thoracic spine
— Fusion operations on the thoracic spine

Principal Anatomical Structures

Spinous process, trapezius muscle, greater rhomboid muscle, latissimus dorsi muscle, thoracolumbar fascia, semispinalis muscle, multifidus muscle, long and short rotator muscles, long and short levator muscles of the ribs, transverse process, rib head, costotransverse ligament, radiate ligament of the head of the rib, vertebral body, pleura; intercostal artery, vein, and nerve.

Positioning and Skin Incisions
(Fig. 203)

The patient is placed in a prone or lateral position; the ipsilateral arm is abducted so as to remove the shoulder-blade from the spine. Pressure on the abdomen should be avoided. When the segment in question has been marked and a radiograph taken, a paramedian skin incision is made in a rectangular shape. Alternatively, hinge-like, arcuate, or straight skin incisions may be employed.

Dissection of the Upper Soft Tissues
(Fig. 204)

The superficial musculature is separated along its median insertion, transected over the rib to be exposed, and retracted superiorly and inferiorly. After exposure of the transverse process, the rib heads and the rib are dissected, the periosteum being retracted.

Dissection in the Osseous Plane
(Fig. 205)

The transverse process is divided with a chisel and detached. The readily visible rib head is now exposed and can be removed. After separation of the outer periosteum, the rib is freed with a rib raspatory and is divided, not too far laterally, and removed. At times, resection of an intercostal nerve may become necessary; no intercostal nerves should be transected at levels T9, T10, or T11, since the accompanying spinal artery cannot be spared with certainty and is indispensable for the blood supply of the spinal cord.

After retraction of the pleura (Fig. 206), the lateral surface of the vertebral body is fully visualized.

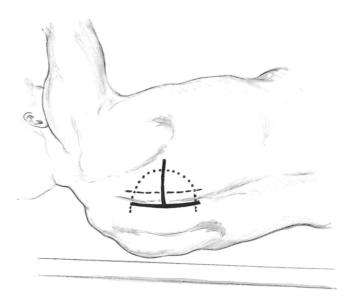

Fig. **203** Lateral approach to the thoracic spine. The patient is placed on the contralateral side, with the arm abducted. The incisions may be longitudinal, arcuate, or like a door (solid line)

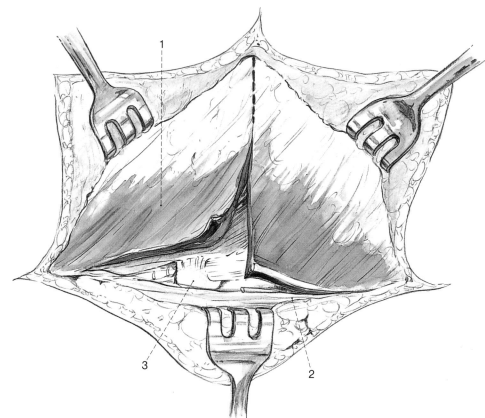

Fig. **204**   Shown here is a T-shaped, door-like skin incision. The trapezius muscle is also divided by a T-incision and elevated. Extension: dashed red line

1   Trapezius muscle
2   Interspinal ligament
3   Transverse process

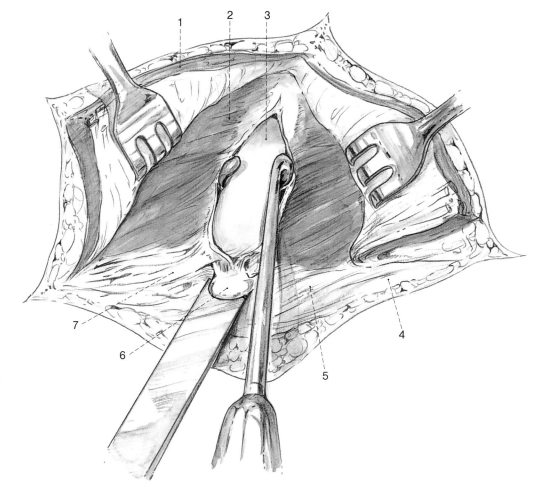

Fig. **205**   The trapezius muscle has been retracted, the outer periosteum of the affected rib longitudinally incised, and the transverse process separated with a chisel. The rib section to be removed is also separated from tissue layers near the lung, so that it can be excised

1   Trapezius muscle
2   External intercostal muscle
3   Rib
4   Supraspinal ligament
5   Interspinal ligament
6   Transverse process
7   Intertransverse ligament

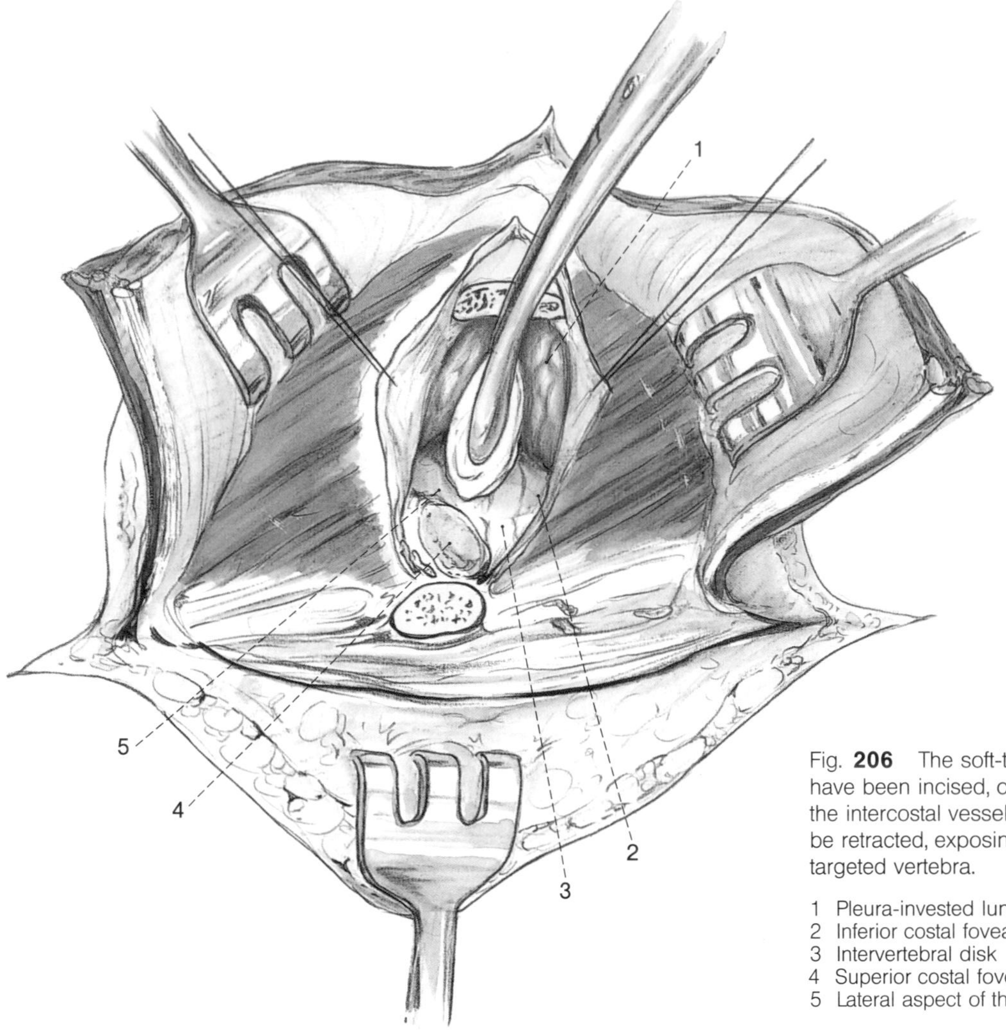

Fig. **206** The soft-tissue layers in the bed of the removed rib have been incised, care being taken to spare the pleura and the intercostal vessels. After this, the pleura-invested lung can be retracted, exposing to view the lateral surface of the targeted vertebra.

1 Pleura-invested lung
2 Inferior costal fovea
3 Intervertebral disk
4 Superior costal fovea
5 Lateral aspect of the vertebral body

Wound Closure

The fascia and the musculature are sutured, a drain is inserted, and the subcutis and cutis are closed. Immediately after the operation, as also on the following days, chest radiographs have to be taken in order to rule out the development of a pneumothorax (pleural injury).

Potential Errors and Dangers

- Hemorrhages from the skin and the soft tissues during the operation
- Injuries to the dura or a nerve, or both
- Pleural injuries, pneumothorax
- Cerebrospinal fluid fistula.

13 Approaches to the Lumbar Spine

Posterior Approach to the Lumbar Spine

Typical Indications for Surgery

— Protrusions and prolapses of the nucleus pulposus
— Stenosis of the lumbar canal
— Tumors
— Vascular malformations

Principal Anatomical Structures

Latissimus dorsi muscle, thoracolumbar fascia, iliocostal and longissimus muscles, interspinal muscles of the loins, long rotatores lumborum muscles, lateral and medial intertransverse muscles of the loins, multifidus muscle, anterior and posterior longitudinal ligaments, lumbar arteries and veins, vertebral venous plexus, spinous processes, vertebral arch, vertebral body, spinal dura mater, spinal medulla, medullary cone, terminal filament, spinal roots, abdominal aorta, inferior vena cava, common iliac artery and vein.

Positioning and Incision
(Figs. 207, 208)

The patient may be placed on his side or in a special prone position (the so-called bunny position). The choice of the position will be decided by the patient's condition, anesthetic requirements, the location of the targeted process, and the surgeon's preferences. In the prone position, provision has to be made for careful padding of all recumbent parts of the body (forehead, arms, knee, instep, toes, etc.). In the lateral position, similar care has to be taken of the arms, knees and ankles.

The incision is made longitudinally; a slightly curved configuration is preferable.

Dissection of the Musculature
(Fig. 209)

The scope of the procedure in the muscular area depends on the extent of the planned exposure at or within the vertebral canal. The length of the incision varies between a very small approach for a fenestration operation in a slim patient, and a considerably longer incision for a laminectomy and for patients with a very strong musculature.

The thoracolumbar fascia is incised with cutting diathermy, and the musculature is retracted subperiosteally with elevators and raspatories. Hemostasis requires monopolar and bipolar coagulation and packing with strips of gauze impregnated with hot saline solution.

Fenestration
(Fig. 210)

With the aid of a special retractor, the medial arm of which is anchored in the lateral surface of the spinous process by a pin, the retracted musculature is removed from the operative field. After separation of the interspinal ligaments, the flaval ligaments are exposed. The approach can be expanded by resecting portions of the arches with fine punches or cooled burrs. The exposed ligamentum flavum is excised or peritomized with a lateral stalk (inset). Below it, nerve roots and the generally targeted alterations of the nucleus pulposus are brought into view.

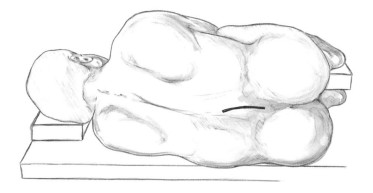

Fig. **207** Posterior approach to the lumbar spine: positioning on the side and incision

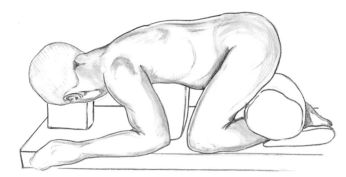

Fig. **208** Posterior approach to the lumbar spine: positioning in the so-called bunny position. The incision is performed as indicated in Figure **207**

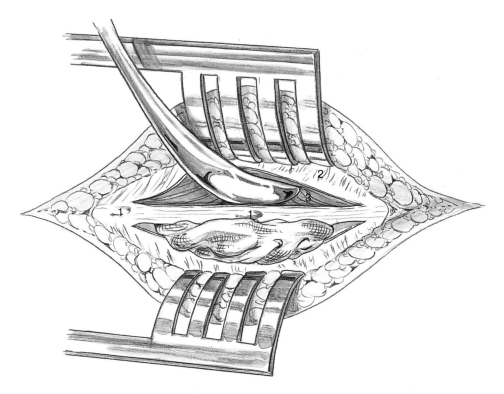

Fig. **209** The skin and the subcutaneous fatty tissue have been distracted. Directly alongside the marked spinous process, the fascia is incised, and the muscle is subperiosteally retracted. For effective reduction of hemorrhages, a gauze strip impregnated with hot saline solution is inserted into the cavity

1 Spinous process
2 Thoracolumbar fascia
3 Iliocostal muscle of loins

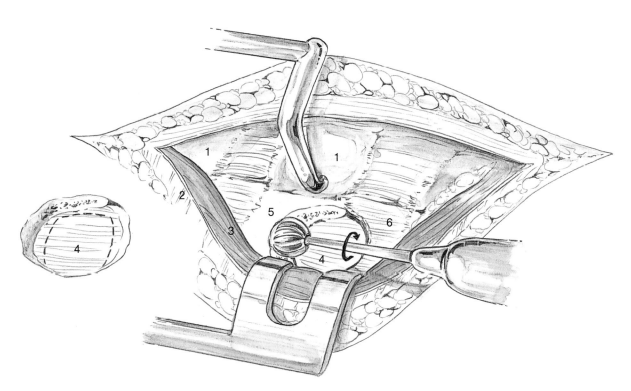

Fig. **210** For a fenestration operation, the musculature is retracted from the spinous process, and the exit site of the marked spinal root is exposed. Adjacent bone is removed with a fine burr if necessary. The exposed ligamentum flavum is incised with a fine knife along the red broken line shown in the inset

1 Spinous process
2 Thoracolumbar fascia
3 Iliocostal muscle of loins
4 Ligamentum flavum
5 Lamina of vertebral arch
6 Interspinal ligament

Hemilaminectomy
(Fig. 211)

A somewhat larger exposure of the intervertebral space is accomplished by removal of the complete lamina of the vertebral arch with fine punches or burrs. The subsequent procedure is unremarkable. In the lumbar region, too, additional space for the operation can be gained by drilling off the medial portions of the spinous process.

Laminectomy
(Fig. 212)

In a complete laminectomy, the interspinal ligaments to the adjacent spinous processes are transected first. After this, the spinous process can be ablated with Luer or Liston bone forceps. Resection of the remaining bone with punches or burrs is the last step. Finally, the epidural adipose tissue is visualized. Small hemorrhages are controlled by bipolar coagulation or by applying hemostatic cloth.

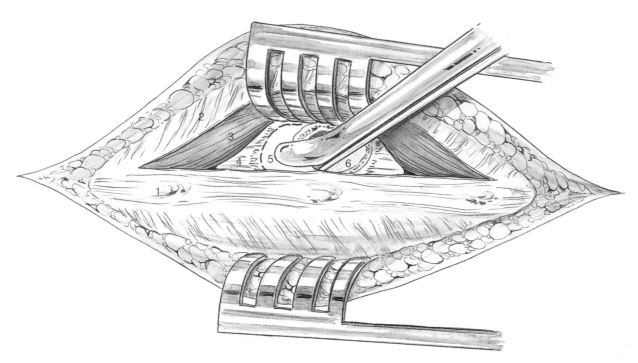

Fig. **211** For a hemilaminectomy, one lamina is removed with punches or burrs. Additional space can be obtained by reaming off the medial base of the spinous process (red dashed line)

1 Spinous process	4 Flaval ligament
2 Thoracolumbar fascia	5 Lamina of vertebral arch
3 Iliocostal muscle of loins	6 Epidural adipose tissue

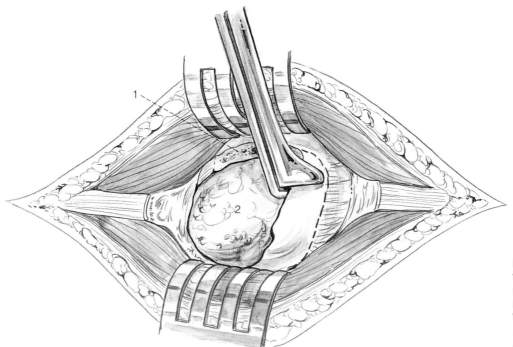

Fig. **212** For a lumbar laminectomy, the spinous process and the adjacent parts of the arch are ablated with punches or burrs. The epidural fatty tissue is visualized (red dashed line)

1 Lamina of vertebral arch (divided)
2 Epidural adipose tissue

Opening the Dura
(Fig. 213)

After elevation of the dura with a fine point, it can be opened longitudinally with knives or scissors. Several dural elevation sutures can be placed to ensure full utilization of the approach. The nerve roots concealed by the arachnoid are now brought into view.

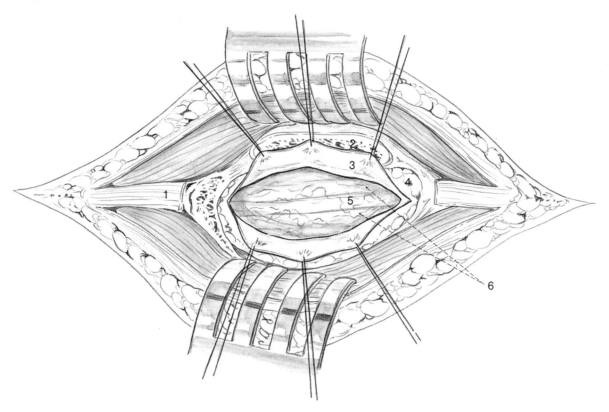

Fig. **213** The dura in the exposed area is longitudinally incised and elevated with sutures. Under the arachnoid, the lumbar spinal roots are brought into view

1 Spinous process	4 Epidural adipose tissue
2 Lamina of vertebral arch	5 Arachnoid
3 Spinal dura mater (elevated by suture)	6 Spinal roots

Wound Closure

If the dura has been opened, it is closed with interrupted or continuous sutures. Epidural hemostasis has to be verified once again.

In the next step, the various muscle layers have to be secured with interrupted sutures, again with careful examination for detection of rebleeding vessels. If necessary in individual cases, a suction drain can be inserted.

The skin is customarily closed with interrupted sutures, though there is no general rule against the use of continuous sutures.

Potential Errors and Dangers

— Overlooked blood loss from soft tissues during the course of the operation
— Failure to reach the targeted vertebral level owing to inadequate marking procedures
— Injury to nerve roots by punches or scissors
— Injury to abdominal vessels
— Insufficient final hemostasis

Posterior Approach to Extracanalicular Regions of the Lumbar Spine

Typical Indications for Surgery

- Extracanalicular disk herniation
- Laterally infiltrating tumors
- Extracanalicularly induced nerve compression

Principal Anatomical Structures

Dorsal process, thoracolumbar fascia, vertebral arch and articulation, interspinal muscles of the loins, longissimus muscle, multifidus muscles, long and short rotator muscles of the loins (spinotransverse system), intervertebral foramen, ligamentum flavum, interspinal ligament, lumbar arteries and veins (dorsal branch), intertransverse muscle, intertransverse ligament, perineural adipose tissue.

Positioning and Skin Incision
(Fig. 214)

In the knee-elbow position, a generally median skin incision is made over the level being targeted and the cranially and caudally adjacent vertebral levels. Also suitable is a paramedian skin incision of equal magnitude performed at a distance of 1–2 cm from the midline. Some surgeons prefer the lateral position, or a tilted, prone, semisitting position.

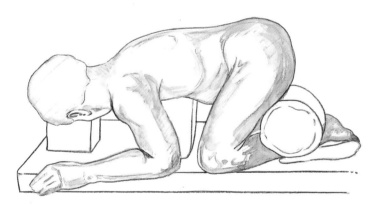

Fig. **214** Posterior approach to extracanalicular intervertebral disk hernias: positioning

Dissection of Soft Tissues
(Fig. 215)

The thoracolumbar fascia is divided on the targeted side about 1.5 cm beside the midline and retracted medially with two holding sutures. The muscle insertions at the spinous process and the vertebral arch are bluntly exposed while sparing the muscle tissue as much as possible, and are divided sharply or with an electric knife. This is followed by meticulous hemostasis at the muscle insertions and the muscle tissue and subsequent coagulation of the dorsal branch of the lumbar artery and vein. The longissimus muscle, with the muscle of the spinotransverse system, is dissected and retracted far enough laterally to expose completely the joint of the affected level as well as the overlying joint with the attachment of the transverse process.

Using a microdrill, the lateral portions of the joint and parts above the joints are ablated (Fig. 216). The intertransverse ligament and the intertransverse muscle are now divided, so that the nerve root in the surrounding fatty tissue can be exposed.

Dissection at the Nerve Root
(Fig. 217)

The surgeon is able to see the lateral opening of the intervertebral canal and also occasionally the cranial portion of the intervertebral disk, and, upon retraction of the surrounding adipose tissue and optical magnification, the nerve root; the latter is usually displaced cranially and dorsally by disk herniation. For removal of subligamentous sequestra, the longitudinal ligament has to be incised as well.

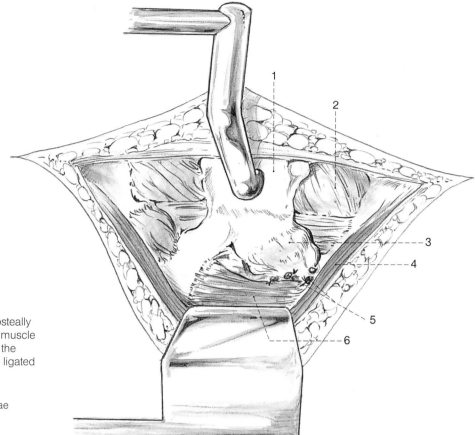

Fig. **215**   The musculature has been extraperiosteally retracted. Vertebral joints and the intertransverse muscle have been exposed, and the dorsal branches of the lumbar artery and vein have been coagulated or ligated

1   Spinous process of the fourth lumbar vertebra
2   Interspinal ligament
3   Articulation of the fourth and fifth lumbar vertebrae
4   Semispinalis lumbalis muscle
5   Lumbar artery and vein (dorsal branch)
6   Intertransverse muscle

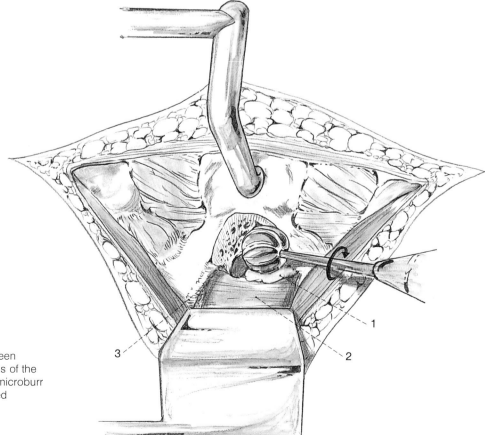

Fig. **216**   The intertransverse muscle has been divided, so that the lateral and cranial portions of the vertebral joint can be ablated with a cooled microburr until the perineural adipose tissue is visualized

1   Perineural adipose tissue
2   Intertransverse ligament
3   Intertransverse muscle (divided)

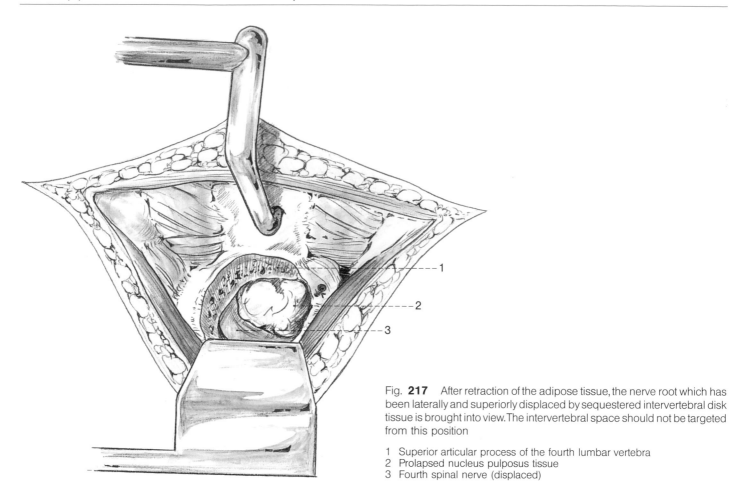

Fig. **217** After retraction of the adipose tissue, the nerve root which has been laterally and superiorly displaced by sequestered intervertebral disk tissue is brought into view. The intervertebral space should not be targeted from this position

1 Superior articular process of the fourth lumbar vertebra
2 Prolapsed nucleus pulposus tissue
3 Fourth spinal nerve (displaced)

Wound Closure

After insertion of a drain in the operative field, the fascia can be closed with interrupted sutures. Layered wound suture completes the operation.

Potential Errors and Dangers

— Faulty localization of the level
— Intraoperative and postoperative hemorrhage due to inadequate hemostasis
— Injury to the nerve root and root sheath
— Incomplete removal of extracanalicularly detected sequestra

14 Approaches to the Peripheral Nervous System

Anterior Approach to the Brachial Plexus

Typical Indications for Surgery

- Blunt injuries (impact, traction, stretching, avulsion)
- Sharp injuries (stab, cut, gunshot)
- Fractures (transverse process, clavicle, first rib, humeral head)
- Dislocations (shoulder joint)

Principal Anatomical Structures

Subclavian muscle, subscapular muscle, smaller pectoral muscle; posterior, middle and anterior scalene muscles; sternocleidomastoid muscle, trapezius muscle, omohyoid muscle, vertebrae, intervertebral foramina, clavicle, first rib, cervical fasciae, vertebral artery, subclavian artery and vein, axillary artery, transverse artery of the neck, thoracic duct.

Positioning and Skin Incision
(Fig. **218**)

The semisitting position with the head turned (and bent) toward the contralateral side has proved satisfactory. The dorsal position, with a firm pad between the shoulderblades and the head, again turned to the contralateral side, is also suitable. The incision begins at the border of the sternocleidomastoid muscle, proceeds toward the middle of the clavicle, traverses the clavicle, and ends in the sulcus of the biceps muscle.

Dissection of the Superficial Supraclavicular Nerves
(Figs. **219, 220**)

The platysma is divided in the direction of the fibers. Situated directly below it are branches from the cervical plexus that run from the border of the sternocleidomastoid muscle toward the clavicle. Next, the superficial cervical fascia and the superficial pectoral fascia are divided. If necessary, the cephalic vein in the clavipectoral trigone and also the external jugular vein are ligated and divided.

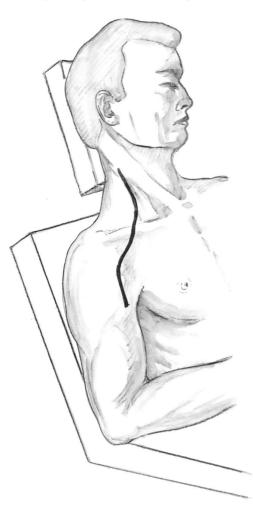

Fig. **218** Exposure of the brachial plexus from the front: positioning and incision

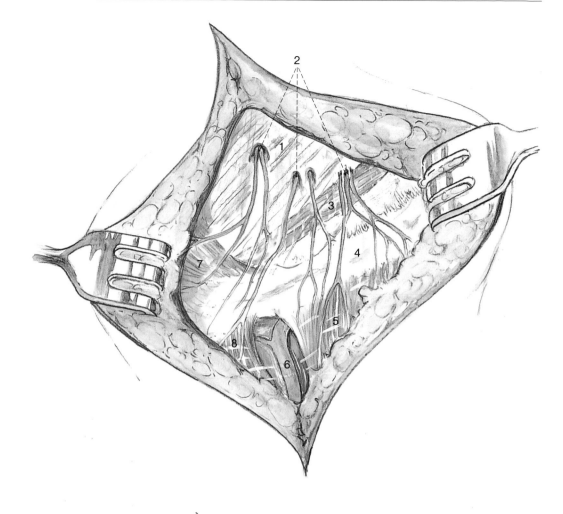

Fig. **219** The skin and the subcutaneous fatty tissue have been distracted with hooks, the platysma has been divided, and the superficial supra-clavicular nerves have been exposed. The main guiding structure is the clavicle

1 Superficial lamina of the cervical fascia
2 Medial, intermediate and lateral supraclavicular nerves
3 Omohyoid muscle (inferior belly)
4 Clavicle
5 Pectoralis major muscle
6 Cephalic vein
7 Trapezius muscle
8 Deltoid muscle

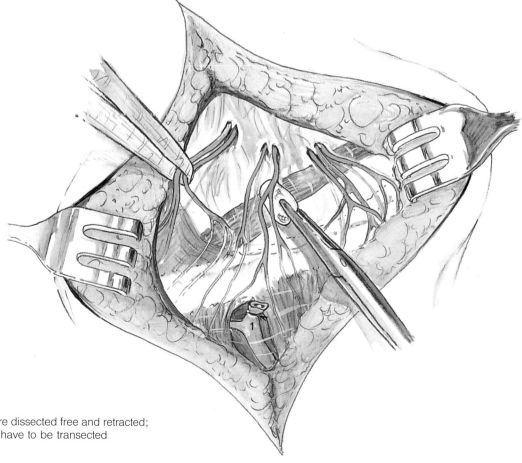

Fig. **220** The supraclavicular nerves are dissected free and retracted; if unavoidable, individual branches may have to be transected

1 Ligated cephalic vein

Division of the Omohyoid Muscle
(Fig. **221**)

In some patients, the exposed omohyoid muscle can be dissected free and then displaced. More commonly, it is divided between ligatures, on which the two parts can subsequently be retracted. Occasionally, it is necessary to notch the clavicular head of the sternocleidomastoid muscle. After these steps, the suprascapular artery is visualized.

Cleavage of the Deep Fascia and Division of the Anterior Scalene Muscle
(Fig. **222**)

The next step involves division of the deep fascia, after which the anterior scalene muscle is brought into view and can be transected. Very close attention should be paid during this procedure to the phrenic and accessory nerves.

Division of the Clavicle
(Fig. **223**)

If the visualization of the brachial plexus is not sufficient, division of the clavicle becomes necessary. For this purpose, the periosteum has to be detached from the middle portion of the clavicle and also from its posterior wall. After this, a gutter-shaped instrument is passed underneath, and the bone over it is divided with a Gigli saw, an oscillating saw, or a similar instrument. The two parts of the bone are then retracted outward from the operative field.

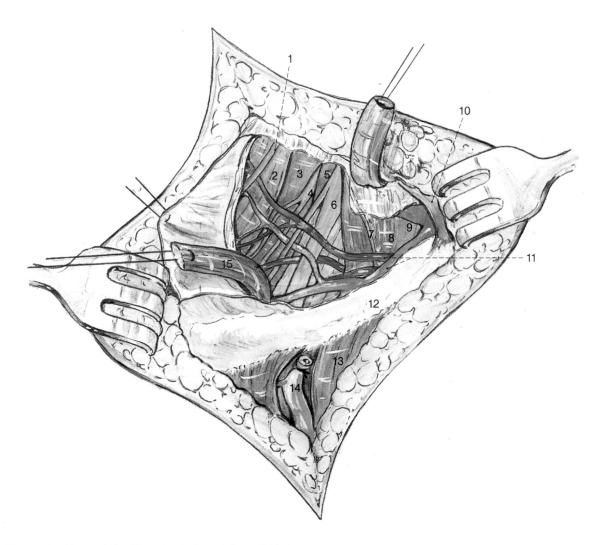

Fig. **221**   The omohyoid muscle is either retracted cranially or divided to permit the deeper structures to be dissected free

1 Accessory nerve	8 Anterior scalene muscle
2 Levator muscle of the scapula	9 Internal jugular vein
3 Posterior scalene muscle	10 Sternocleidomastoid muscle
4 Dorsal nerve of the scapula and long thoracic nerve	11 Suprascapular artery and vein
5 Middle scalene muscle	12 Clavicle
6 Superior trunk	13 Pectoralis major muscle
7 Phrenic nerve	14 Cephalic vein (ligated)
	15 Omohyoid muscle (divided, distal part)

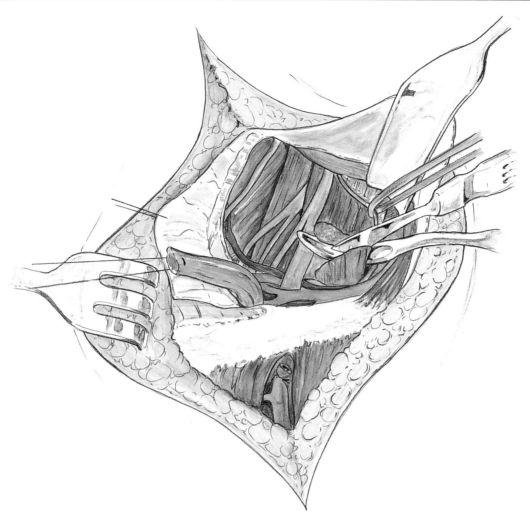

Fig. **222**   For further exposure of the brachial plexus in its supraclavicular segment, division of the anterior scalene muscle may be required. The phrenic nerve coursing on the muscle then has to be isolated, and special care has to be taken to protect it

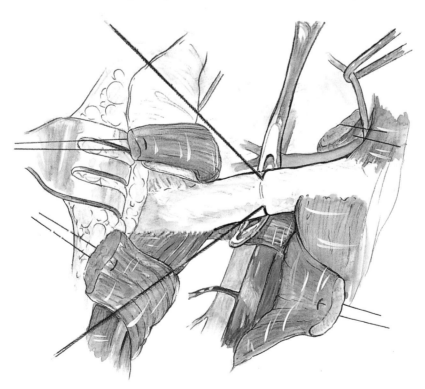

Fig. **223**   If further exposure of the brachial plexus is to be achieved, division of the clavicle becomes necessary (e.g., with the Gigli saw). For this purpose, the vessels adjoining its medial surface need to be retracted. Division of the bone has to be performed on a solid support

Complete Exposure of the Brachial Plexus
(Fig. 224)

Following several blunt dissections, the brachial plexus now lies exposed. Its organization is shown in the illustration. Dissection of the plexus parts can be a time-consuming operative step after blunt local injuries.

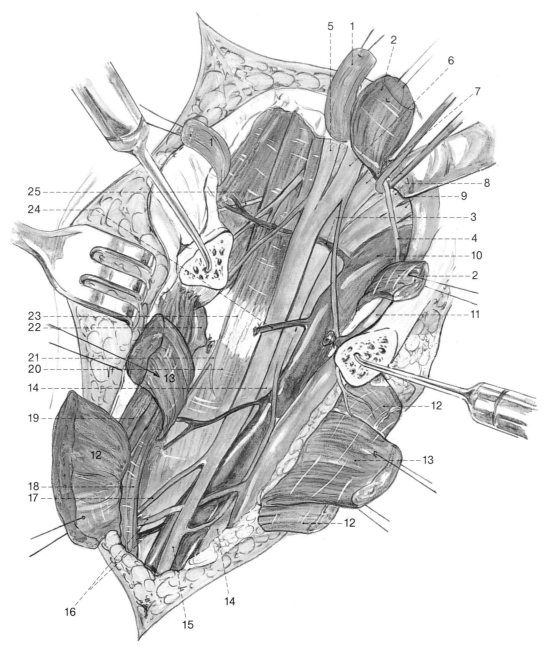

Fig. **224** Distraction of the two parts of the clavicle provides a full view of the vessels and nerves of the axillary fossa

1 Omohyoid muscle
2 Anterior scalene muscle
3 Transverse cervical artery
4 Phrenic nerve
5 Anterior branch of the fifth cervical nerve (C5)
6 Anterior branch of the sixth cervical nerve (C6)
7 Anterior branch of the seventh cervical nerve (C7)
8 Anterior branch of the eighth cervical nerve (C8)
9 Anterior branch of the first thoracic nerve (T1)
10 Subclavian artery
11 Subclavian vein
12 Pectoralis major muscle
13 Pectoralis minor muscle
14 Medial cord

15 Lateral cord
16 Deep brachial artery and vein
17 Musculocutaneous nerve
18 Coracobrachial muscle
19 Deltoid muscle
20 Anterior serratus muscle
21 Long thoracic nerve
22 Cephalic vein
23 First rib
24 Thoracoacromial artery
25 Dorsal nerve of the scapula

Osteosynthesis of the Clavicle

The restoration of continuity and stability of the clavicle at the end of the operation may necessitate consultation with an experienced bone surgeon. The method used for this synthesis is left up to the surgeon's discretion. In addition to wire-suturing, medullary nailing, closure with AO plates, and many other methods can be employed.

Wound Closure

In deeper layers, only divided muscles should be reunited. This type of closure is not necessary in the fascial layers. The subcutaneous and cutaneous sutures are placed and tied individually. The cosmetic outcome should be carefully considered.

Potential Errors and Dangers

— Inadequate ability of the skin incision to expand, due to inadequate incision planning
— Avoidable injury of adjacent vessels and nerves
— Pleural injury
— Development of pseudarthrosis
— Local postoperative hematoma
— Inadequate approximation of the subcutis and skin

Transaxillary Approach to the Brachial Plexus

Typical Indications for Surgery

— A special indication is nerve interposition between the intercostal nerves and the upper arm nerves after avulsion of the brachial plexus
— The causes of avulsions have been described above.

Principal Anatomical Structures

Anterior and middle scalene muscles, subclavian artery and vein, first rib, cervical pleura, anterior serratus muscle.

Positioning and Skin Incision
(Fig. 225)

The patient is placed in a slightly turned-back lateral position, and the arm, bent at the elbow, is pulled upward as far as is possible in the presence of contractures. On the whole, the position of the arm during the operation should remain mobile. The slightly concave skin incision is made in the axilla at the border with the thorax, between the borders of the latissimus dorsi and the greater pectoral muscles; if necessary, it can be extended in a curve toward the upper ribs.

Exposure of Muscles in the Axillary Funnel
(Fig. 226)

To begin with, the fatty tissue within the axilla can be dissected laterally; some of it has to be removed. After this, the greater pectoral muscle at the superior wound margin can be mobilized and retracted cranially. The lower portions of the brachial plexus, as well as the vessels, now enter the field of vision. They lie on the surface formed by the brachial biceps, latissimus dorsi, and subscapular muscles. Underneath, the anterior serratus muscle and the thorax are brought into view.

Exposure of Other Parts of the Plexus and Communicating Nerves
(Fig. 227)

In the next step, the operative field can be widened and deepened. This requires separating the communicating nerves in the area of the thoracic wall and preparing them for anastomoses. Alongside the portions of the plexus, the dissection can be extended deeper into the axillary funnel; however, the approach becomes very narrow, and is associated with a risk of additional pressure-induced and traction-induced lesions of the plexal parts.

Wound Closure

Notched muscles have to be sutured. The closure of the subcutis and skin is carried out in accordance with cosmetic considerations, taking account especially of the delicate skin of the axilla and the course of the incision, which promotes cicatricial contraction.

Potential Errors and Dangers

— Injury to additional vessels and nerves, particularly the thin epithoracic structures
— Pleural injury
— Stretch and pressure lesions due to overly vigorous use of spatulas
— Local postoperative hematomas due to inadequate hemostasis

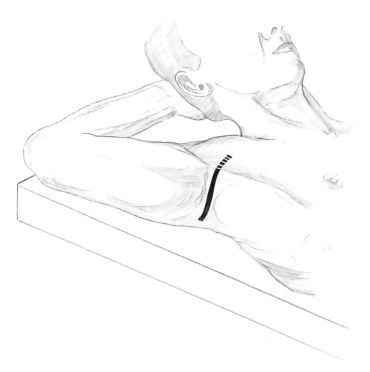

Fig. **225** Axillary approach to parts of the brachial plexus: positioning and incision

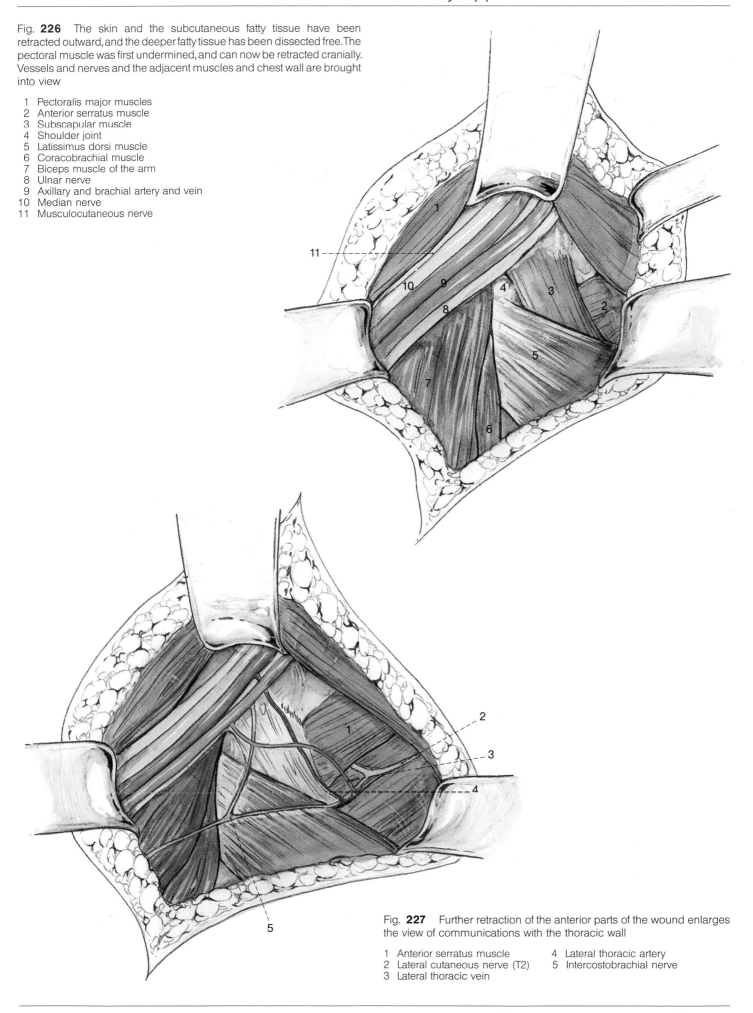

Fig. **226** The skin and the subcutaneous fatty tissue have been retracted outward, and the deeper fatty tissue has been dissected free. The pectoral muscle was first undermined, and can now be retracted cranially. Vessels and nerves and the adjacent muscles and chest wall are brought into view

1 Pectoralis major muscles
2 Anterior serratus muscle
3 Subscapular muscle
4 Shoulder joint
5 Latissimus dorsi muscle
6 Coracobrachial muscle
7 Biceps muscle of the arm
8 Ulnar nerve
9 Axillary and brachial artery and vein
10 Median nerve
11 Musculocutaneous nerve

Fig. **227** Further retraction of the anterior parts of the wound enlarges the view of communications with the thoracic wall

1 Anterior serratus muscle
2 Lateral cutaneous nerve (T2)
3 Lateral thoracic vein
4 Lateral thoracic artery
5 Intercostobrachial nerve

Approach to the Accessory Nerve

For clinical reasons, the treatment of related injuries of the accessory nerve is described at this point even though this is not a peripheral but a cranial nerve.

Typical Indications for Surgery

— Sharp injuries (stab, cut, gunshot)
— Blunt injuries (kick, hematoma)
— Iatrogenic injury during removal of lymph nodes from the lateral cervical triangle, e.g., in tuberculosis

Principal Anatomical Structures

Jugular vein, sternocleidomastoid and trapezius muscles, lymph nodes of the lateral cervical triangle, accessory nerve, lesser occipital nerve, and greater auricular nerve.

Positioning and Skin Incision
(Fig. 228)

The patient is in a supine position, with the head turned to the opposite side. The skin incision parallels the upper third of the posterior border of the sternocleidomastoid.

Identification of Adjacent Nerves
(Fig. 229)

Three adjacent nerves are found in this region. The lesser occipital nerve has a much thinner trunk, and does not give off any branches. The great auricular nerve runs in the direction of the auricular region. The accessory nerve maintains its course from above to inferior-posterior.

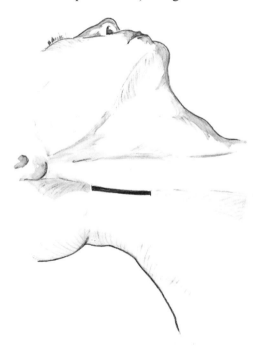

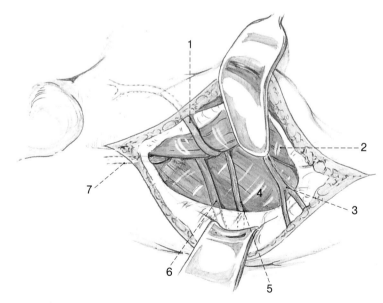

Fig. **228** Approach to the accessory nerve in the lateral cervical triangle: positioning and incision. The guiding structure is the posterior border of the sternocleidomastoid muscle

Fig. **229** The accessory nerve and surrounding structures have been exposed

1 Great auricular nerve
2 Sternocleidomastoid muscle
3 Lateral supraclavicular nerve
4 Anterior scalene muscle
5 Trapezius branch
6 Accessory nerve
7 Lesser occipital nerve

Wound Closure

The subcutis and the adipose tissue are resutured on the basis of cosmetic considerations.

Potential Errors and Dangers

— Injury to additional nerves
— Local postoperative hematomas due to inadequate hemostasis

Approach to the Axillary Nerve

Typical Indications for Surgery

— Sharp injuries (cut, stab, gunshot)
— Blunt injuries
— Fractures (humeral head, scapula)
— Dislocations (shoulder joint)
— Iatrogenic lesions (reduction, shoulder surgery)

Principal Anatomical Structures

Subscapular muscle, radial nerve and axillary artery, posterior circumflex humeral artery and vein, teres major and triceps muscles, humerus, deltoid muscle.

Positioning and Skin Incision
(Fig. 230)

The patient is placed in a decidedly overdrawn lateral position, with the hand of the affected side resting on the contralateral shoulder joint. The skin incision begins in the middle of the superior border of the scapula and continues along the border of the deltoid muscle.

Incision of Soft Tissues
(Fig. 231)

To begin with, the fascia has to be divided. Hereafter, the deltoid muscle may be retracted superiorly. The dissection requires special care because of the immediately adjacent vessels.

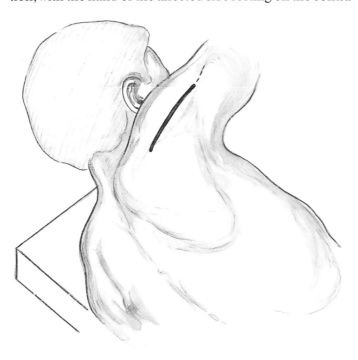

Fig. 230 Exposure of the axillary nerve in the shoulder region: positioning and incision. The deltoid muscle is the guiding structure

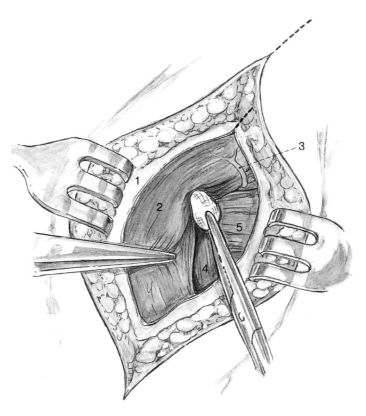

Fig. 231 After the superficial fascia has been split, the deltoid and teres major muscles are retracted from the long head of the triceps muscle, visualizing, to begin with, a branch of the superior lateral cutaneous nerve of the arm. *Red dashed lines:* possible extensions

1 Deltoid fascia
2 Deltoid muscle
3 Branch of superior lateral cutaneous nerve of the arm
4 Teres minor muscle
5 Triceps muscle of arm (long head)

Dissection of Nerve

(Fig. 232)

The surrounding vessels include particularly the posterior circumflex humeral artery. The nerve itself lies in the angle between the teres minor muscle and the long head of the triceps muscle.

Wound Closure

Fascial sutures are not generally needed. The subcutis and the cutis are sutured according to cosmetic requirements.

Potential Errors and Dangers

— Insufficient enlargement of the skin incision due to inadequate planning of its location
— Injury of vessels close to the humerus
— Overextension of nerves due to excessive spatula traction
— Postoperative local hematomas due to inadequate hemostasis

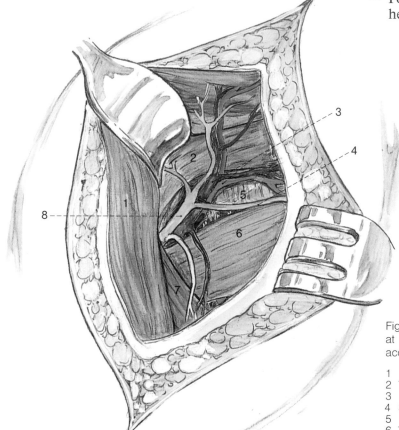

Fig. **232**   Deeper extension of the wound gives access to the nerve at the cranial border of the latissimus dorsi muscle and to the accompanying posterior circumflex humeral artery

1 Deltoid muscle
2 Triceps muscle of arm (lateral head)
3 Posterior circumflex humeral artery and vein
4 Superior lateral cutaneous nerve of the arm
5 Latissimus dorsi muscle
6 Triceps muscle of the arm (long head)
7 Teres minor muscle
8 Axillary nerve, with division into the anterior and posterior branches

Approach to the Musculocutaneous Nerve

Typical Indications for Surgery

— Sharp injuries (stab, cut, gunshot)
— Blunt injuries (kick, traction, hematoma)
— Fracture (very rare; humeral shaft)
— Iatrogenic injuries (injections)

Principal Anatomical Structures

Greater pectoral muscle, subscapular tendon, median nerve, medial border of coracobrachial muscle, brachial muscle, biceps muscle of arm, and brachioradial muscle.

Positioning and Skin Incisions at Various Levels
(Fig. 233)

The patient is in a supine position; the arm is abducted at right angles and rotated outward. The skin incisions run along the border of the deltoid muscle and around the border of the greater pectoral muscle into the axilla and then into the medial bicipital sulcus.

Exposure in the Axilla
(Fig. 234)

The greater pectoral muscle is divided a few centimeters anterior to its insertion; after this the brachial biceps muscle can be retracted and the underlying neurovascular bundle exposed.

Exposure in the Upper Third of the Upper Arm
(Fig. 235)

Dissection along the border of the greater pectoral muscle is at first carried in a distal direction; after this, the fascia can be divided and the biceps muscle of the arm retracted laterally. This exposes the brachial muscle. The musculocutaneous nerve lies laterally inside the visible neurovascular bundle.

Exposure in the Lower Third of the Upper Arm
(Fig. 236)

After the division of the brachial fascia, the brachial biceps and brachial muscles are visualized. When these two muscles are distracted, the neurovascular bundle is once again exposed.

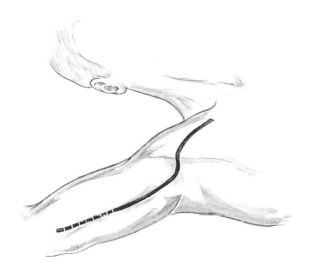

Fig. **233** Exposure of the musculocutaneous nerve in the axillary and upper arm regions: positioning and incision in the medial bicipital sulcus

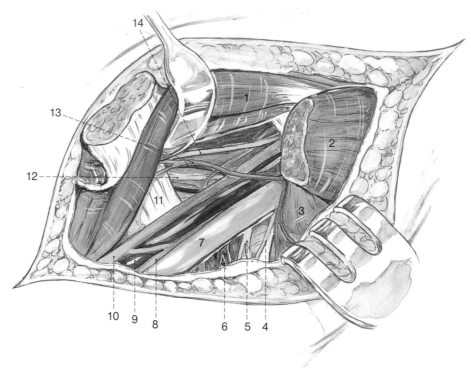

Fig. **234** In the area of the axilla, the neurovascular tract is visualized after division of the pectoral muscle and lateral displacement of the biceps muscle

1 Biceps muscle of the arm (long and short heads)
2 Pectoralis major muscle (divided)
3 Pectoralis minor muscle
4 Long thoracic nerve
5 Thoracodorsal nerve
6 Circumflex artery of scapula
7 Axillary vein

8 Ulnar nerve
9 Axillary artery
10 Median nerve
11 Latissimus dorsi muscle
12 Axillary nerve
13 Posterior circumflex humeral artery and vein
14 Musculocutaneous nerve

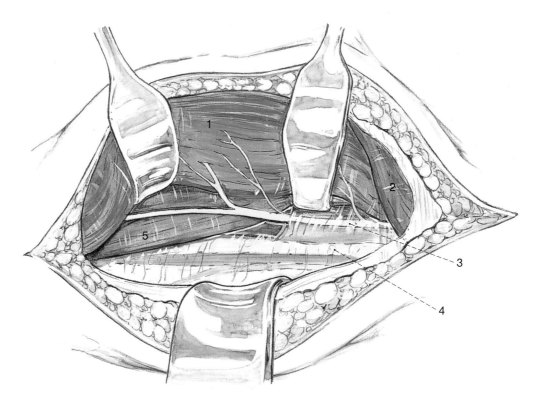

Fig. **235** In the upper third of the upper arm, the dissection proceeds, after division of the deep fascia, between the short head of the biceps muscle of the arm and the coracobrachial muscle and continues on the brachial muscle, with the neurovascular bundle adjoining medially

1 Biceps muscle of the arm (short head)
2 Deltoid muscle
3 Musculocutaneous nerve
4 Neurovascular bundle
5 Brachial muscle

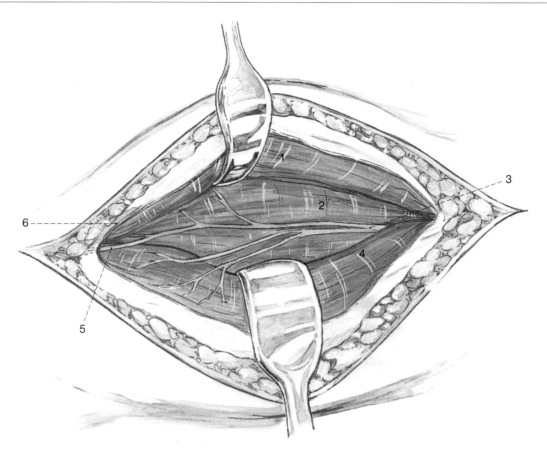

Fig. **236** In the lower third of the upper arm, the dissection is performed between the biceps muscle of the arm and the triceps muscle. On the brachial muscle, additional muscle branches and the lateral cutaneous nerve of the forearm are split off

1 Biceps muscle of arm
2 Brachial muscle
3 Musculocutaneous nerve
4 Triceps muscle of the arm
5 Lateral cutaneous nerve of the forearm
6 Cephalic vein

Wound Closure

Divided muscles are reunited. Occasionally, the approximation of a thick fascia becomes necessary. The subcutaneous tissue and the skin are closed in accordance with cosmetic considerations.

Potential Errors and Dangers

— Injury to additional nerves due to instruments and over-extension
— Injury to vessels
— Local postoperative hematomas due to inadequate hemostasis

Approaches to the Median Nerve

Typical Indications for Surgery

- Sharp injuries (stab, cut, gunshot)
- Blunt injuries (pressure, traction, hematoma)
- Fractures (humeral head, humeral shaft, supracondylar humeral fracture, distal radial fracture)
- Dislocations (elbow)
- Iatrogenic injuries (reduction of fractures and dislocations, plaster cast, osteosyntheses, injections, wound care, ischemia)
- Compression (carpal tunnel, supracondylar, aponeurosis musculi bicipitis brachii – formerly termed lacertus fibrosus)

Principal Anatomical Structures

Tendon of the greater pectoral muscle, subscapular muscle, shoulder joint capsule, musculocutaneous nerve, axillary artery, axillary vein, ulnar nerve, biceps muscle of the arm and brachial muscle, pronator teres muscle, deep flexor muscle of the fingers and long flexor muscle of the thumb, carpal tunnel, palmar aponeurosis.

Positioning and Skin Incisions

(Fig. **237**)

Axilla. The patient is in a supine position; the upper arm is fully abducted, while the lower arm is flexed and the palm placed below the occiput; the ipsilateral thorax is elevated. The slightly convex skin incision runs deep in the axilla from the greater pectoral muscle to the latissimus dorsi muscle and may, if necessary, be extended at right angles to the biceps muscle of the arm.

Upper arm. The arm of the supine patient is rectangularly abducted and externally rotated. The skin incision extends in the medial bicipital sulcus from the border of the pectoral muscle to the elbow; it can, of course, be shorter. The basilic vein should be kept in sight.

Elbow. The patient is again supine, with the arm abducted at right angles, and the forearm supinated. The skin incision (Fig. **238**) is Z-shaped, running from the medial bicipital sulcus across the elbow, and then vertically along the ulnar border of the brachioradial muscle. Attention should be paid to the basilic and cephalic veins.

Forearm. The positioning is as above, with the arm resting on a side table. The skin incision (Fig. **239**) extends from the middle of the elbow to the middle of the flexor side of the forearm.

Wrist. The position conforms to the two descriptions above. The course of the skin incision has a double-S shape course (Fig. **240**), circling the ball of the thumb, traversing the wrist, and continuing ulnarly on the distal forearm.

Dissection of the Neurovascular Bundle in the Axilla

(Fig. **241**)

After division of the fascia, the short head of the biceps and the coracobrachial muscle can be exposed and retracted laterally. After this, the borders of both the greater pectoral and the latissimus dorsi muscles have to be identified and pulled apart. From the skin to the depth, the neurovascular bundle emerges in the following order: axillary vein, musculocutaneous nerve, axillary artery, median nerve.

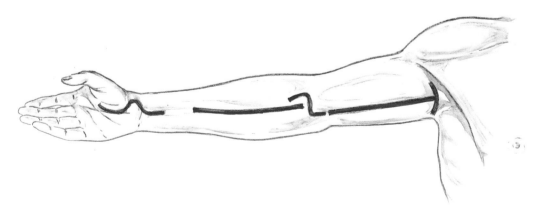

Fig. **237** Exposure of the median nerve: positioning and incisions (beware of joints)

Fig. **238** Z-shaped incision for exposure of the median nerve in the region of the elbow

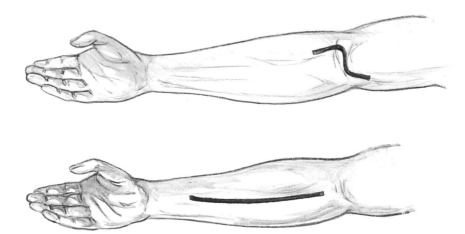

Fig. **239** Incision for exposure of the median nerve in the forearm

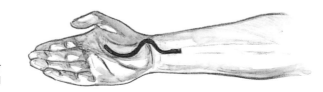

Fig. **240** Incision in the shape of a double S for exposure of the median nerve in the area of the carpal tunnel

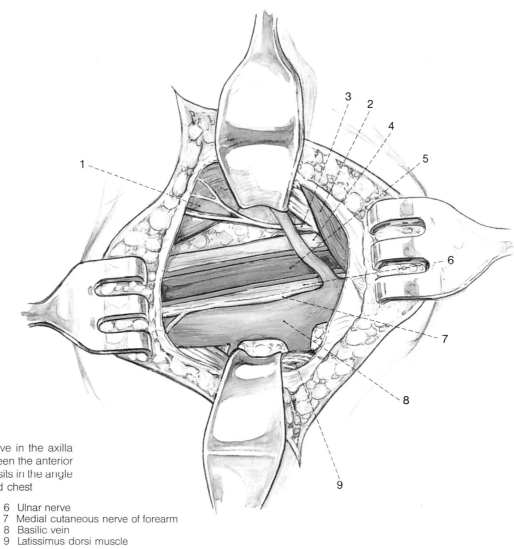

Fig. **241** Exposure of the median nerve in the axilla after transverse incision of the skin between the anterior and posterior axillary folds. The surgeon sits in the angle between the patient's abducted arm and chest

1 Coracobrachial muscle
2 Greater pectoral muscle
3 Musculocutaneous nerve
4 Median nerve
5 Brachial artery with concomitant veins
6 Ulnar nerve
7 Medial cutaneous nerve of forearm
8 Basilic vein
9 Latissimus dorsi muscle

Dissection of the Neurovascular Bundle in the Upper Arm
(Fig. 242)

The brachial fascia is first divided along the medial border of the biceps muscle of the arm; after this, the muscle can be retracted laterally, exposing the neurovascular bundle (from the skin to the depth: musculocutaneous nerve, median nerve, brachial artery, medial cutaneous nerve of the forearm, brachial vein, ulnar and radial nerves). From the middle of the upper arm, the median nerve crosses the brachial artery.

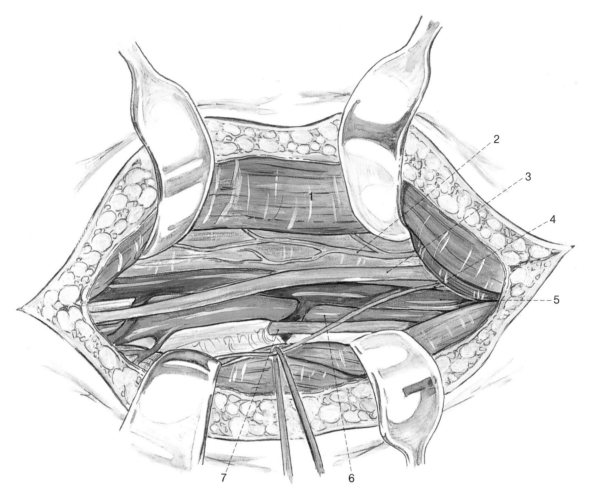

Fig. **242**   In the region of the upper arm, the median nerve is exposed between the biceps and triceps muscles of the arm. It is visualized above the readily palpable brachial artery and, along its further course, it crosses the artery

1 Biceps muscle of the arm
2 Musculocutaneous nerve
3 Median nerve
4 Medial cutaneous nerve of the forearm
5 Brachial artery and accompanying vein
6 Basilic vein
7 Ulnar nerve

Dissection of the Neurovascular Bundle at the Elbow
(Fig. 243)

The fascia is incised vertically, and the lacertus fibrosus is transected. The pronator teres muscle can then be retracted medially, and the brachioradial and the long and short extensor muscles of the wrist can be retracted laterally. The median nerve lies on the brachial muscle and the biceps tendon. The nerve, accompanied by the brachial artery, runs between the heads of the pronator teres muscle.

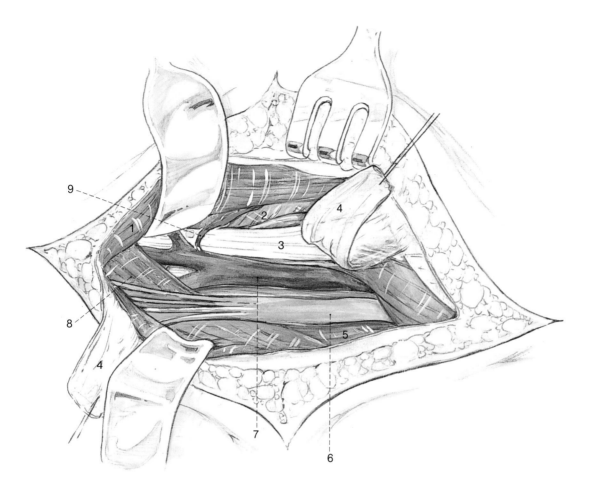

Fig. **243**   For dissection of the median nerve at the elbow, the aponeurosis of the biceps muscle of the arm (lacertus fibrosus) is divided, and the brachioradial muscle is displaced laterally, so that the vessels and nerves can be exposed

1 Brachioradial muscle
2 Supinator muscle
3 Biceps muscle of the arm
4 Aponeurosis of the biceps muscle of the arm (lacertus fibrosus, divided)
5 Brachial muscle
6 Median nerve
7 Brachial artery
8 Pronator teres muscle
9 Radial recurrent artery

Dissection of the Neurovascular Bundle of the Forearm

(Figs. 244–246)

To begin with, the lacertus fibrosus is divided so that the brachioradial muscle can be retracted laterally and the pro- nator teres muscle can be retracted medially. The brachial artery gives off the radial artery, and thus divides into the ulnar and common interosseous arteries. In some cases, the radial insertion of the pronator teres muscle and, occasion- ally, that of the flexor muscle of the fingers as well, has to be separated.

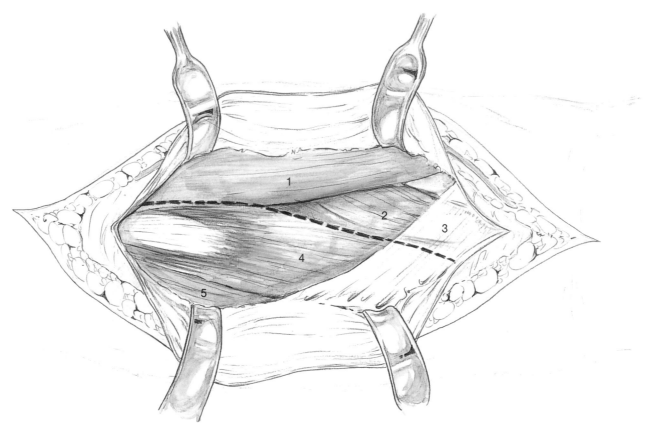

Fig. **244**   For exposure of the median nerve in the forearm, the superfi- cial fascia is divided, and an incision is started between the brachioradial muscle and the radial flexor muscle of the wrist and continued in the direc- tion of the elbow at the border of the radial flexor muscle of the wrist; in addition, the aponeurosis of the biceps muscle of the arm (lacertus fibro- sus) is transected

1 Brachioradial muscle
2 Pronator teres muscle
3 Aponeurosis of the biceps muscle of the arm (lacertus fibrosus)
4 Radial flexor muscle of the wrist
5 Long palmar muscle

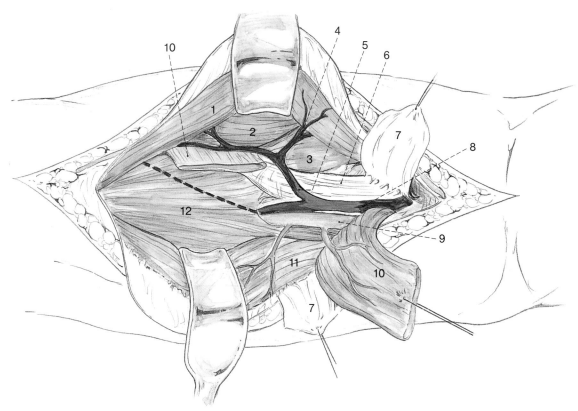

Fig. **245** In the next step, the brachioradial muscle and the radial flexor muscle of the wrist can be retracted, so that the teres pronator muscle can be obliquely transected. The vessels and nerves are visualized below. The superficial flexor muscle of the fingers, which has also been exposed, can be divided if necessary at a small angle to the direction of its fibers

1 Brachioradial muscle
2 Long radial extensor muscle of the wrist
3 Supinator muscle
4 Radial recurrent artery
5 Radial artery
6 Tendon of the biceps muscle of the arm
7 Aponeurosis of the biceps muscle of the arm (lacertus fibrosus)

8 Brachial artery
9 Median nerve
10 Pronator teres muscle
11 Radial flexor muscle of the wrist
12 Superficial flexor muscle of the fingers, with incision line

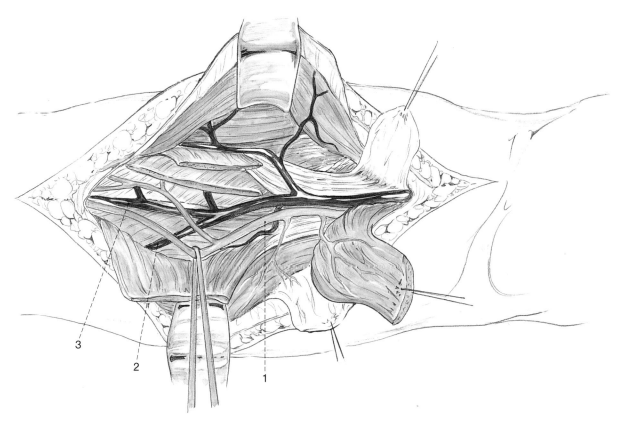

Fig. **246** Division of the superficial flexor muscle of the fingers has brought into view the further course of nerves and vessels

1 Median nerve
2 Ulnar artery
3 Anterior interosseous artery

183

Dissection of the Neurovascular Bundle of the Wrist
(Fig. 247)

The main task is the successive longitudinal division of the retinaculum of the flexor muscles on the ulnar side. The palmar branch of the median nerve in particular, as well as the local vessels, have to be spared.

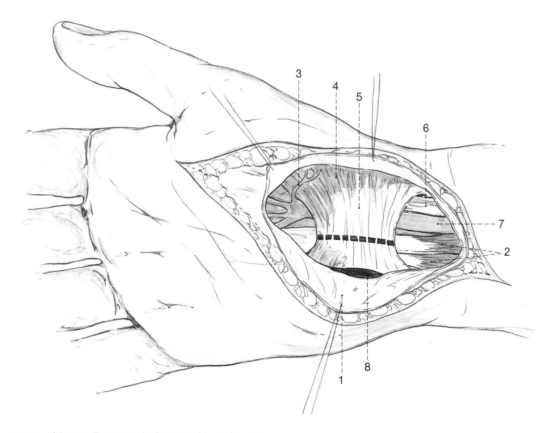

Fig. **247** For exposure of the median nerve in the carpal tunnel, numerous types of incision have been proposed; the skin incision should not be made too small. The division of the flexor retinaculum is performed on the ulnar side in order not to injure the nerve and, above all, its muscular branch

1 Palmar aponeurosis
2 Superficial flexor muscle of the fingers
3 Muscular branch of median nerve
4 Short abductor and flexor muscle of the thumb
5 Flexor retinaculum, with incision line
6 Radial flexor muscle of the wrist
7 Median nerve
8 Ulnar artery

Wound Closure

Notched and divided muscles are resutured. The fasciae require such sutures only occasionally. The closure of subcutaneous tissues and the skin is guided by cosmetic considerations.

Potential Errors and Dangers

– Added damage to vessels and nerves due to instruments, overextension and pressure
– Insufficient consideration of cosmetic aspects during wound closure
– Local postoperative hematomas due to inadequate hemostasis

Approaches to the Radial Nerve

Typical Indications for Surgery

— Sharp injuries (cut, gunshot)
— Blunt injuries (pressure, traction, impact, hematoma)
— Sequelae of fractures (humeral head, humeral shaft, supracondylar humeral fracture, fractures of radial heads or shaft, wrist bone)
— Iatrogenic (operative treatment of fractures, adjacent surgery, positioning, plaster cast, ischemia)

Principal Anatomical Structures

Subscapular muscle, teres major muscle, latissimus dorsi muscle, axillary artery, axillary nerve, median and ulnar nerves, brachial artery, humeral shaft, triceps muscle of the arm, brachial and brachioradial muscles, short supinator muscle, pronator teres muscle, superficial flexor muscle of the fingers, radial artery, radial shaft, interosseous membrane, neck of the radius, extensor group, radiocarpal joint.

Positioning and Skin Incisions

Upper third of upper arm (Fig. **248**): Supine or lateral position, with the palm resting on the contralateral shoulder and the upper arm underpadded. The skin incision proceeds at the posterior border of the deltoid muscle in the direction of the lateral epicondyle.

Middle third of upper arm: Same positioning as above. The longitudinal incision follows the acromion-olecranon apex line, or else the incision is made in the extension of the aforementioned incision and continues to the lateral border of the biceps.

Lower third of upper arm: Same position as above. The skin incision is made in the lateral bicipital sulcus and extends maximally as far as the intersection with the radial extensor muscle of the wrist.

Superficial branch (Fig. **249**): Same position as above, with supinated and adducted arm. The skin incision is made in the lateral bicipital sulcus, bypasses the lateral epicondyle, and continues on the long radial extensor muscle of the wrist.

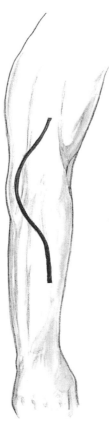

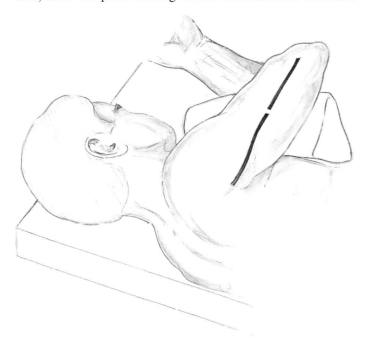

Fig. **248** Exposure of the radial nerve in the upper arm, at the elbow, and in the forearm. For the operation on the upper arm, the patient lies on the side with the underpadded and angulated arm drawn forward; for the more distal operations, the arm is abducted and made to rest on a separate table. The surgeon now sits between the patient's arm and chest

Fig. **249** Incision around the epicondyle for exposure of the superficial branch of the radial nerve

Deep branch (Fig. **250**): With the patient supine, the arm is abducted by 45 degrees and the forearm is moderately flexed. The skin incision is placed in the lateral bicipital sulcus in the direction of the lateral epicondyle, or in the groove between the long radial extensor muscle of the wrist and the extensor muscle of the fingers, in the direction of the middle finger.

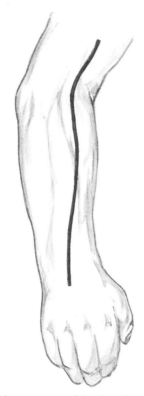

Fig. **250**   Incision for exposure of the deep branch of the radial nerve

Exposure of the Nerve in the Upper Third of the Upper Arm
(Fig. **251**)

In the first step, the fascia of the deltoid muscle is incised, the muscle is retracted medially, and the area of the triceps heads is exposed. The latter may then be separated. By this means the teres major muscle is visualized; immediately below its inferior border, the radial nerve, accompanied by the deep brachial artery, is brought into view.

Exposure of the Nerve in the Middle Third of the Upper Arm
(Fig. **252**)

When the brachial fascia has been longitudinally incised, both the radial nerve and the deep brachial artery are visualized between the medial and lateral heads of the triceps muscle of the arm.

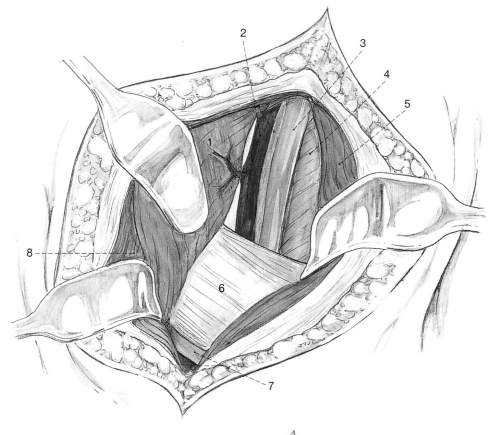

Fig. **251** In the proximity of the shoulder, the massive lateral and long heads of the triceps muscle of the arm and the deltoid muscle first have to be drawn apart in order to visualize the vessels and nerves

1 Triceps muscle of the arm (lateral head)
2 Deep brachial artery and vein
3 Radial nerve
4 Triceps muscle of the arm (medial head)
5 Triceps muscle of the arm (long head)
6 Teres major muscle
7 Posterior circumflex humeral artery and vein
8 Deltoid muscle

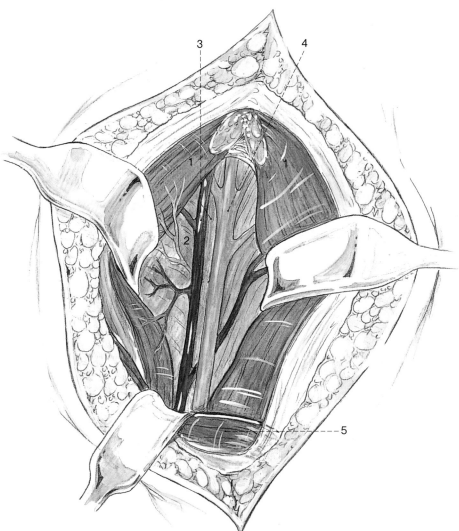

Fig. **252** In the middle third of the upper arm, dissection proceeds via the triceps muscle of the arm (long head), with an added incision if need be. The vessels being sought, and the radial nerve, lie below

1 Triceps muscle of the arm (long head)
2 Triceps muscle of the arm (lateral head)
3 Deep brachial artery and vein
4 Radial nerve
5 Teres major muscle

Exposure of the Nerve in the Lower Third of the Upperarm

(Fig. 253)

After the skin incision, the cephalic vein and the lateral cutaneous nerve of the arm have to be observed and spared.

Division of the fascia makes possible the medial retraction of the lateral border of the biceps muscle. After this, the border of the brachioradial muscle can be exposed, allowing the muscle to be retracted laterally; at this site, attention has to be paid to the musculocutaneous nerve and the lateral cutaneous nerve of the forearm.

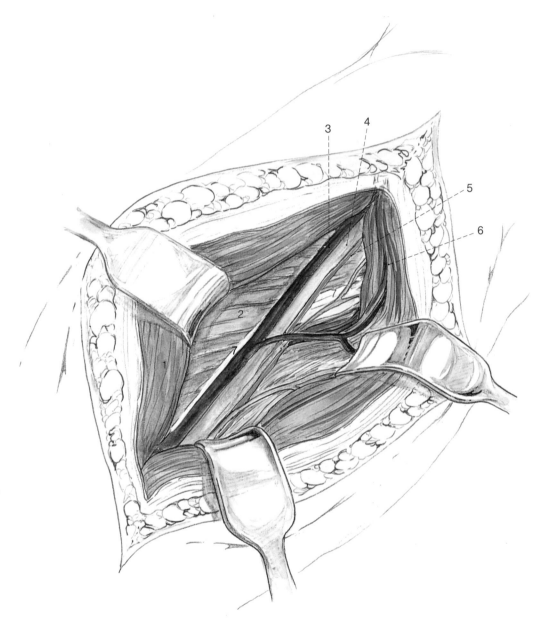

Fig. **253**   In the lower third of the upper arm, the lateral and long heads of the triceps muscle are retracted, so that once again the nerve and the vessels are brought into view

1 Triceps muscle of the arm (lateral head)
2 Triceps muscle of the arm (medial head)
3 Deep brachial artery
4 Radial nerve
5 Deep brachial vein
6 Triceps muscle of the arm (long head)
7 Humerus

Exposure of the Superficial Branch in the Forearm

(Fig. 254)

Initially, the antebrachial fascia is incised. After this, the medial border of the brachioradial muscle can be dissected and the muscle retracted laterally. The radial nerve and artery course on the anterior surface of the supinator muscle and on the surface of the pronator teres muscle.

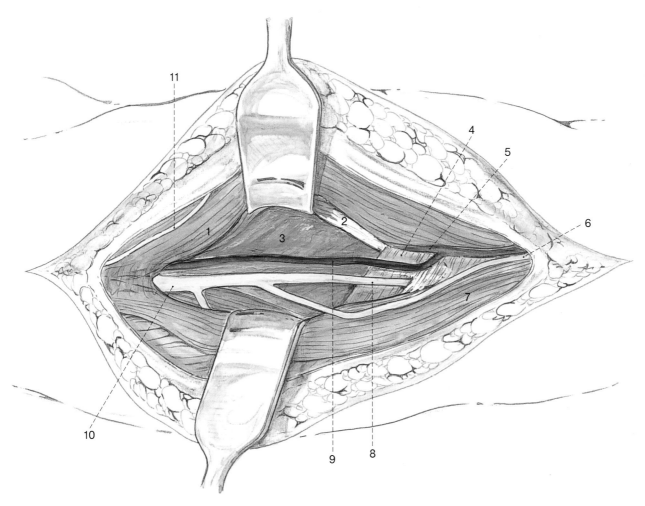

Fig. **254** For exposure of the superficial branch of the radial nerve, the biceps muscle of the arm and the brachioradial muscle have to be drawn apart. The nerve and vessels on the brachial muscle can be brought into view

1 Biceps muscle of the arm
2 Biceps tendon
3 Brachial muscle
4 Supinator teres muscle
5 Radial artery
6 Superficial branch of the radial nerve
7 Brachioradial muscle
8 Deep branch of the radial nerve
9 Radial recurrent artery
10 Radial nerve
11 Lateral cutaneous nerve of the forearm

Exposure of the Deep Branch in the Forearm
(Fig. 255)

Again, the antebrachial fascia has to be incised first. Subsequently, the radial extensor muscle of the wrist can be retracted radially. The deep branch pierces the supinator muscle. Care is required in dissecting the branches for the extensor group.

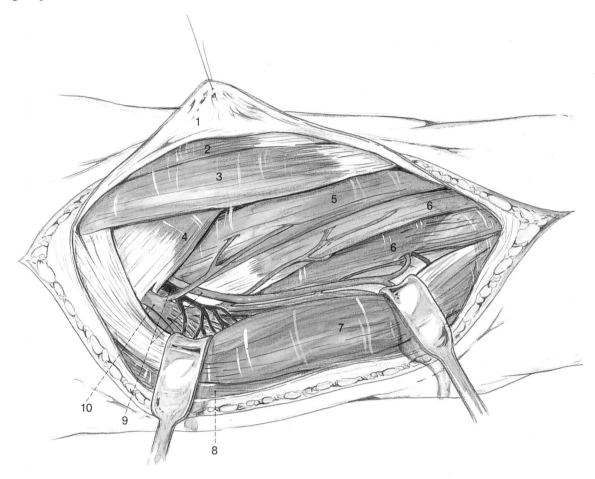

Fig. **255** For exposure of the deep branch of the radial nerve, the extensor muscle of the fingers is retracted in an ulnar direction

1 Antebrachial fascia
2 Long radial extensor muscle of the wrist
3 Short radial extensor muscle of the wrist
4 Supinator muscle
5 Long abductor muscle of the thumb
6 Long and short extensor muscle of the thumb
7 Extensor muscle of the fingers
8 Ulnar extensor muscle of the wrist
9 Posterior interosseous artery and vein
10 Deep branch of the radial nerve

Wound Closure

Notched and divided muscles are rejoined by suture. Thicker portions of fascia also have to be reunited. The subcutaneous tissue and the skin should be closed in accordance with cosmetic considerations, special care being taken over joints to avert the formation of contractile scars.

Potential Errors and Dangers

— Injury to adjacent vessels and nerves
— Pressure and traction lesions of contiguous nerves due to overly vigorous application of spatulas
— Local postoperative hematomas due to inadequate hemostasis
— Unsatisfactory cutaneous scar formation

Approaches to the Ulnar Nerve

Typical Indications for Surgery

— Sharp injuries (glass, knife, gunshot)
— Blunt injuries (pressure, traction, impact, hematoma)
— Sequelae of fractures (humerus, ulna)
— Sequelac of dislocations
— Cubital tunnel syndrome
— Late paralysis of ulnar nerve
— Iatrogenic (operative treatment of fractures, removal of tumors and lymph nodes, positioning, plaster cast, ischemia)

Principal Anatomical Structures

Axillary artery and vein, median nerve, radial nerve, greater and smaller pectoral muscles; subscapular, teres major, latissimus dorsi, coracobrachial and brachial biceps muscles; brachial artery, medial bicipital sulcus, medial epicondyle, olecranon, sulcus of ulnar nerve, ulnar flexor muscle of the wrist and superficial flexor muscle of the fingers, ulnar artery, flexor retinaculum, pisiform bone.

Positioning and Skin Incisions

The patient is generally placed in a supine position, with the upper arm abducted rectangularly and the forearm flexed and supinated. On the upper arm (Fig. 256), the incision is made in the medial bicipital sulcus; on the elbow (Fig. 257), it is made directly over the medial epicondyle or (preferably) around the epicondyle. On the forearm, the skin incision runs a straight or wavy course from the medial epicondyle to the pisiform bone (the radial border of the ulnar flexor muscle of the wrist), while the exposure on the wrist uses an S-shaped incision that curves around the hypothenar prominence and the pisiform bone (Fig. 258). For the last two exposures, it is advantageous to rest the arm on a separate table next to the actual operating table.

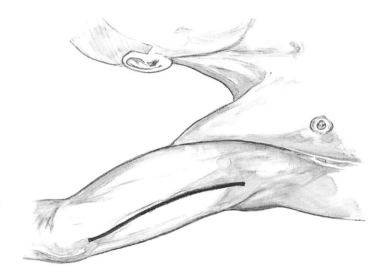

Fig. **256** Exposure of ulnar nerve at various levels. The arm is abducted and rests on a separate table. The surgeon sits between the patient's arm and chest

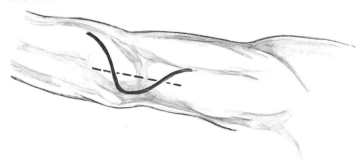

Fig. **257** Incision for exposure of the ulnar nerve at the elbow. *Dashed line:* for short exposure

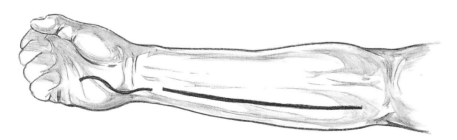

Fig. **258** Incision for exposure of the ulnar nerve in the forearm and hand

Exposure of the Nerve in the Upper Arm
(Fig. **259**)

Initially, the medial border of the biceps muscle of the arm is dissected, after which the brachial fascia is incised and, finally, the biceps muscle of the arm is retracted anteriorly and the triceps muscle posteriorly. The neurovascular bundle is now exposed: musculocutaneous nerve, median nerve (strongest nerve), brachial artery and vein, ulnar nerve, upper third of radial nerve; border of biceps, median nerve, brachial artery and vein, ulnar nerve, triceps muscle of the arm in the middle and lower thirds of the upper arm.

Exposure of the Nerve at the Elbow Level
(Fig. **260**)

Here the skin incision follows transection of the superficial layer of the collateral ulnar ligament and then of the arch connecting the two origins of the ulnar flexor muscle of the wrist. After this, the neurovascular bundle is exposed.

Exposure of the Nerve in the Forearm
(Fig. **261**)

First, the radial border of the ulnar flexor muscle of the wrist is dissected; the other boundary of the medial antebrachial sulcus is formed by the superficial flexor muscle of the fingers. In this way, the nerve lying on the deep flexor muscle of the fingers and accompanied by the ulnar artery is visualized.

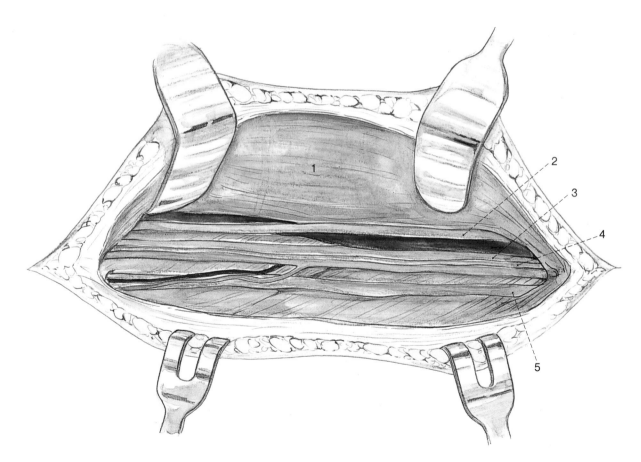

Fig. **259** Exposure of the ulnar nerve in the upper arm requires radial displacement of the biceps muscle, so that vessels and nerves can be visualized

1 Biceps muscle of the arm
2 Median nerve
3 Brachial artery and vein
4 Medial cutaneous nerve of the forearm
5 Ulnar nerve

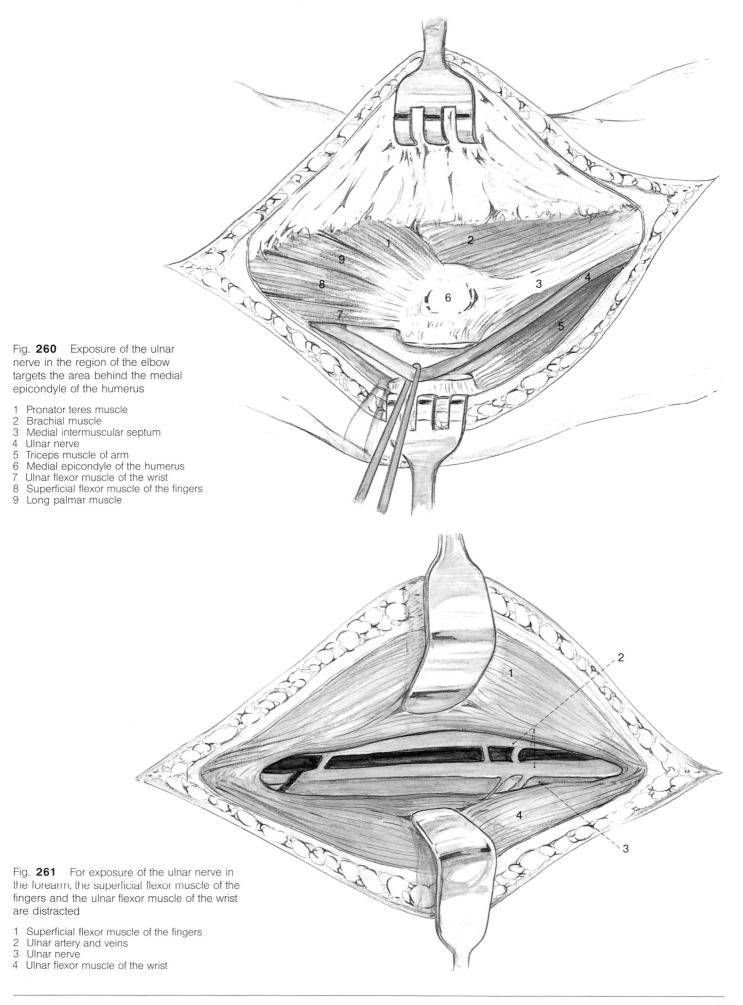

Fig. **260** Exposure of the ulnar nerve in the region of the elbow targets the area behind the medial epicondyle of the humerus

1 Pronator teres muscle
2 Brachial muscle
3 Medial intermuscular septum
4 Ulnar nerve
5 Triceps muscle of arm
6 Medial epicondyle of the humerus
7 Ulnar flexor muscle of the wrist
8 Superficial flexor muscle of the fingers
9 Long palmar muscle

Fig. **261** For exposure of the ulnar nerve in the forearm, the superficial flexor muscle of the fingers and the ulnar flexor muscle of the wrist are distracted

1 Superficial flexor muscle of the fingers
2 Ulnar artery and veins
3 Ulnar nerve
4 Ulnar flexor muscle of the wrist

Exposure of the Nerve at the Wrist

(Fig. 262)

Following the skin incision, the antebrachial fascia is split in a longitudinal direction, and so is the flexor retinaculum, more distally. Whether incision of the palmar aponeurosis and the short palmar muscle also becomes necessary depends on the exact location of the lesion and the extent of the exposure.

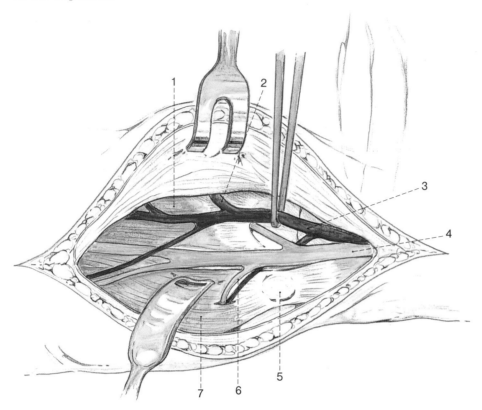

Fig. 262 Exposure of the ulnar nerve in the area of the wrist is guided by the palpable and visible pisiform bone

1 Short flexor muscle of the little finger
2 Deep branch of the ulnar artery
3 Ulnar artery
4 Ulnar nerve
5 Pisiform bone
6 Nerves and vessels for the hypothenar musculature
7 Abductor muscle of the little finger

Wound Closure

Transected and notched muscles are rejoined; thick fasciae are sutured. Subcutaneous tissue and the skin require closure in accordance with cosmetic considerations.

Potential Errors and Dangers

— Damage to adjacent vessels and nerves due to instruments and pressure and traction from spatulas
— Local postoperative hematomas due to inadequate hemostasis
— Cosmetic problems in wound healing

Approach to the Ilioinguinal Nerve

Typical Indications for Surgery

— Idiopathic ilioinguinal neuralgia
— Painful states following herniotomy, renal, and ureteral surgery

Principal Anatomical Structures

Greater psoas muscle, quadratus lumborum muscle, transverse muscle of the abdomen, internal oblique muscle of the abdomen, iliac crest, anterior superior iliac spine, inguinal ligament.

Positioning and Skin Incision

(Fig. 263)

The patient is placed in a supine position, and the pelvis is elevated on the side to be operated on. The skin incision is made 2 cm above the lateral and medial thirds of the inguinal ligament.

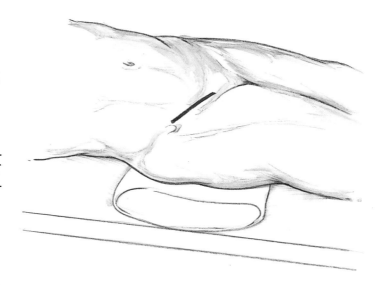

Fig. **263**   Exposure of the ilioinguinal nerve in the inguinal region: positioning and incision above the inguinal ligament

Dissection of Soft Tissues

(Fig. 264)

Next, the aponeurosis of the external oblique muscle of the abdomen is incised, and the round ligament of the uterus (spermatic cord) is dissected.

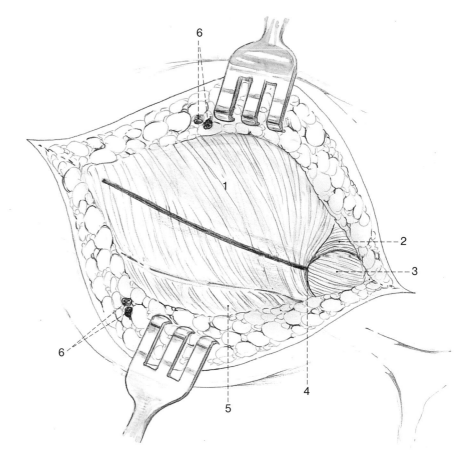

Fig. **264**   To begin with, the aponeurosis of the external oblique muscle of the abdomen is opened parallel to the inguinal ligament, and thus parallel to the inguinal canal

1 Aponeurosis of the external oblique muscle of the abdomen
2 Medial inguinal crus
3 Spermatic cord
4 Lateral inguinal crus
5 Inguinal ligament
6 Superficial epigastric artery and vein

Exposure of the Nerve
(Fig. **265**)

The nerve passes through the abdominal musculature and then takes an oblique course, similar to that of the muscle fibers, in a medial-inferior direction. It lies in the inguinal canal, lateral and caudal to the teres uteri ligament (spermatic cord), between the aponeuroses of the external oblique and internal (i.e. cremasteric) muscles of the abdomen.

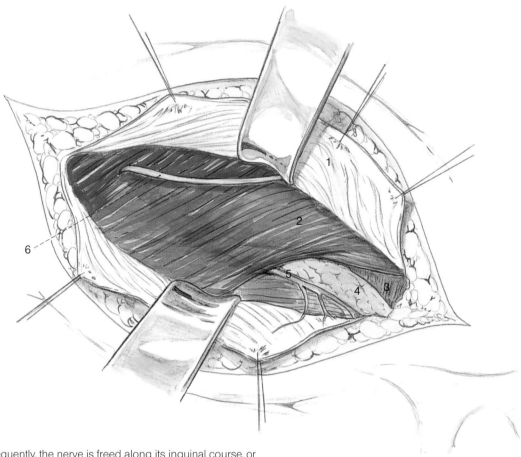

Fig. **265**   Subsequently, the nerve is freed along its inguinal course, or else can be dissected free from local scars

1   Aponeurosis of the external oblique muscle of the abdomen
2   Internal oblique muscle of the abdomen
3   Reflected ligament
4   Spermatic cord
5   Ilioinguinal nerve
6   Iliohypogastric nerve

Wound Closure

After closure of the oblique muscle aponeurosis, the subcutaneous tissues and the skin may be sutured, taking account of cosmetic requirements.

Potential Errors and Dangers

— Injuries to the spermatic cord
— Excessive constriction of the spermatic cord during suture of aponeuroses
— Local postoperative hematoma due to inadequate hemostasis

Approaches to the Genitofemoral Nerve

Typical Indications for Surgery

— Idiopathic genitofemoral neuralgia
— Neuralgia secondary to appendectomy, herniotomy, etc.

Principal Anatomical Structures

Greater psoas muscle, retroperitoneal adipose tissue, common and external iliac arteries, inguinal ligament, lacuna vasorum, femoral artery.

Positioning and Skin Incisions

(Fig. 266)

The patient is placed in a supine position; the operative side of the back is elevated so that the body arches upward.

The oblique incision runs from the costal margin (median axillary line) to the umbilicus. The optional longitudinal incision takes a ventrolateral course, that is, one analogous to the skin incision for exposure of the lumbar sympathetic trunk.

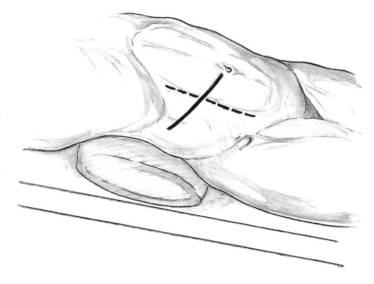

Fig. **266** Exposure of the genitofemoral nerve in the abdominal region: positioning and incisions. The following figures represent the cross incision (solid line). *Dashed incision lines:* adipose tissue.

Dissection of Soft Tissues

(Fig. 267)

To begin with, the fibers of the external oblique muscle of the abdomen are distracted; after this, the aponeurosis of the muscle can be divided. In the next step, the fibers of the internal oblique muscle and the transverse muscle of the abdomen have to be distracted to permit incision of the transverse fascia. Particular attention should be paid at this point to the peritoneum. The viscera can now be retracted with drapes and long spatulas, and finally the iliopsoas muscle can be exposed.

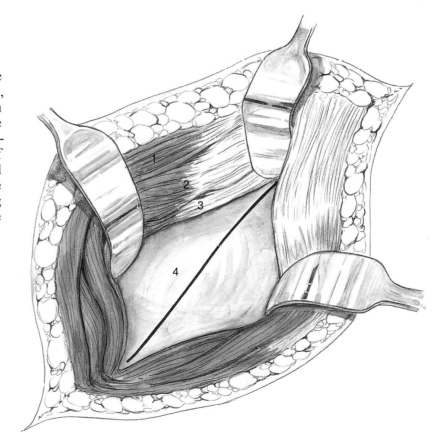

Fig. **267** Following layered separation of the external abdominal musculature, the transverse fascia is reached. It is incised along the line shown here (straight or wavy line)

1 External oblique muscle of the abdomen
2 Internal oblique muscle of the abdomen
3 Transverse muscle of the abdomen
4 Transverse fascia

Exposure of the Nerve
(Fig. **268**)

In the procedure on the right side of the body, it is necessary to retract the inferior vena cava medially. Now exposed, the genitofemoral nerve runs obliquely, from superior-lateral to inferior-medial, to the medial border of the muscle. More medially, both the lumbar sympathetic trunk and the junctions of the transverse processes with the vertebral bodies are visualized.

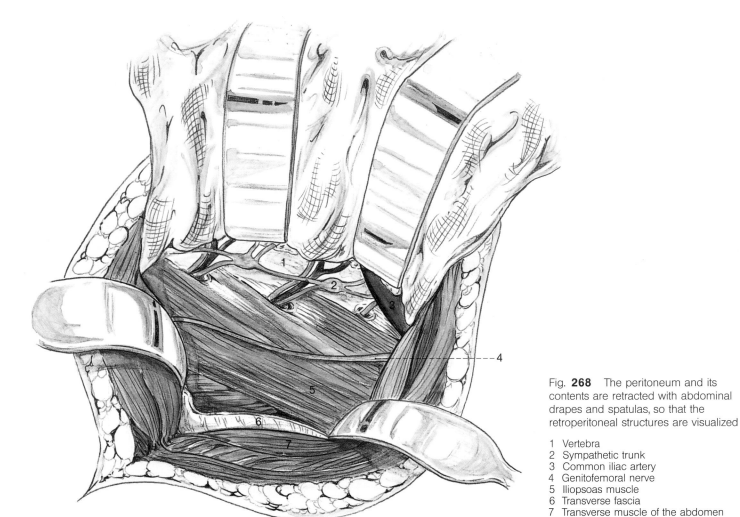

Fig. **268** The peritoneum and its contents are retracted with abdominal drapes and spatulas, so that the retroperitoneal structures are visualized

1 Vertebra
2 Sympathetic trunk
3 Common iliac artery
4 Genitofemoral nerve
5 Iliopsoas muscle
6 Transverse fascia
7 Transverse muscle of the abdomen

Wound Closure

The oblique and transverse muscles are closed again; this may require some muscle-approximation sutures. Finally, the subcutaneous tissues and the skin are carefully sutured.

Potential Errors and Dangers

— Overlooked injuries to the peritoneum
— Overlooked injuries to the inferior vena cava
— Postoperative hemorrhages from other sources
— Abdominal hernias due to inadequate suture of fasciae

Approach to the Lateral Cutaneous Nerve of the Thigh

Typical Indications for Surgery

— Meralgia paresthetica
— Harvesting of interposition material

Principal Anatomical Structures

Ala ossis ilii, iliac muscle, cecum (right), and sigmoid (left), deep circumflex iliac artery, inguinal ligament, fascia lata, origin of sartorius muscle, anterior superior iliac spine.

Positioning and Skin Incision
(Fig. 269)

The operation is performed with the patient in a supine position and the buttocks slightly raised on the affected side. A skin incision 7–8 cm long is made 3 cm below and parallel to the lateral third of the inguinal ligament, or one centimeter inward from the anterior superior iliac spine in the longitudinal direction of the leg. The length of the incision depends on the amount of subcutaneous fat in this area, and is thus markedly shorter in slim patients.

Dissection of Soft Tissues
(Fig. 270)

The fascia lata is split parallel and close to the inguinal ligament, and the remaining part is dissected upward in the direction of the inguinal ligament. Enlargement of the exposure may necessitate a more or less extensive notching of the sartorius muscle insertion.

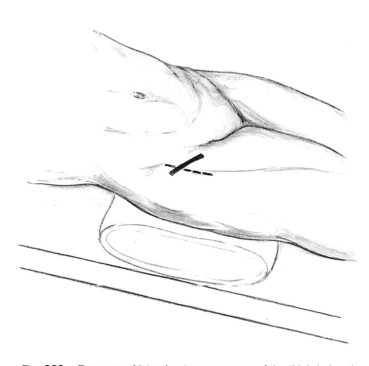

Fig. **269** Exposure of lateral cutaneous nerve of the thigh below the inguinal ligament: positioning and incisions. In the figures below, an incision parallel to the inguinal ligament is shown

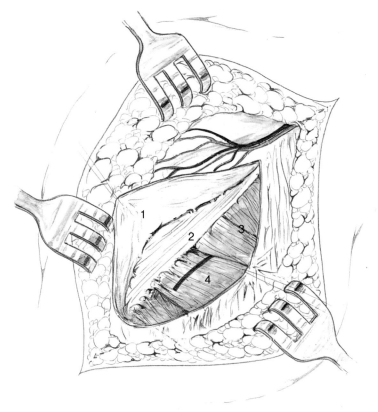

Fig. **270** After opening of the fascia lata, the sartorius muscle can be notched

1 Fascia lata
2 Inguinal ligament
3 Iliopsoas muscle with divergent directions of the fibers
4 Sartorius muscle, with incision line marked

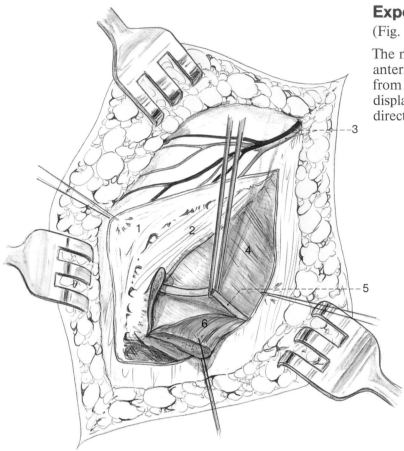

Exposure of Nerve
(Fig. **271**)

The nerve enters the operative field directly medial to the anterior superior iliac spine. It runs a slightly oblique course from superior-lateral to inferior-medial. If it is merely to be displaced, blunt and sharp dissection is carried out in both directions.

Fig. **271** The notching brings into view the lateral cutaneous nerve of the thigh

1 Fascia lata
2 Inguinal ligament
3 Superficial circumflex iliac artery and vein
4 Iliopsoas muscle
5 Lateral cutaneous nerve of the thigh
6 Sartorius muscle (incised and reflected)

Wound Closure

The fascia lata and the notched sartorius muscle are closed by suture. Closure of subcutaneous tissues and the skin according to cosmetic requirements completes the operation.

Potential Errors and Dangers

— Damage to adjacent nerves and vessels
— Inadequate closure of the fascia lata

Approaches to the Femoral Nerve

Typical Indications for Surgery

- Hip joint operations (endoprostheses, femoral neck nailing, osteotomy)
- Gynecologic operations (spatula pressure)
- Herniotomy, appendectomy
- Vascular reconstruction in the aortic-iliac region
- Fracture of superior branch of pubic bone
- Hematomas of psoas in coagulation disorders

Principal Anatomical Structures

Greater psoas muscle and iliac muscle, iliac fascia, external iliac artery, inguinal ligament, lacuna of muscles, femoral artery and vein, quadriceps muscle of thigh, great saphenous vein.

Positioning and Skin Incisions
(Fig. 272)

The patient is supine, and the buttocks are underpadded on the affected side. For a procedure in the pelvic region, the leg is internally rotated. In the inguinal region, the skin is incised longitudinally in the middle of the thigh, beginning at the level of the inguinal ligament. However, the incision may also be started over the lateral third of the inguinal ligament; it then describes a curve before continuing vertically. If the operation that damaged the nerve was performed only a short time previously, the skin incision of the first operation is chosen.

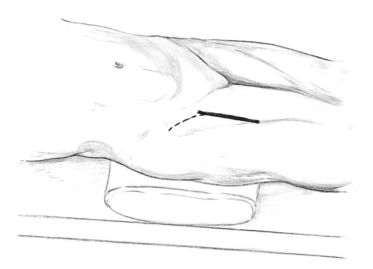

Fig. **272** Exposure of femoral nerve, in the thigh and retroperitoneally (dashed line): positioning and incisions

In the pelvic region, an incision is made a fingerbreadth inward from the medial border of the ventral segments of the ala ossis ilii, and is continued as far as the line connecting the umbilicus with the superior iliac spine.

Dissection of Soft Tissues
(Fig. 273)

After identification of the inguinal ligament, the lymph nodes are retracted from the operative field. The exposed fascia lata is best opened by a T-shaped incision, with the individual T-bars heading medially. This leads to the groove between the iliac muscle and the psoas muscle, which contains vessels and the nerve.

Medially to the iliac crest, the fibers of the external oblique muscle of the abdomen are bluntly divided, and those of the internal oblique muscle and the transverse muscle of the abdomen are transected. After this, the iliac fascia is incised. Following retraction of the extraperitoneal adipose tissue, the peritoneum is retracted medially with drapes and long spatulas.

Exposure of Nerve in Inguinal Region
(Fig. 274)

After careful retraction of the investing femoral vein and artery, the femoral nerve can be dissected free, close attention being paid to its branches. This is particularly important during longitudinal incision of the iliac fascia. In the presence of central lesions, the dissection is carried toward and below the inguinal ligament.

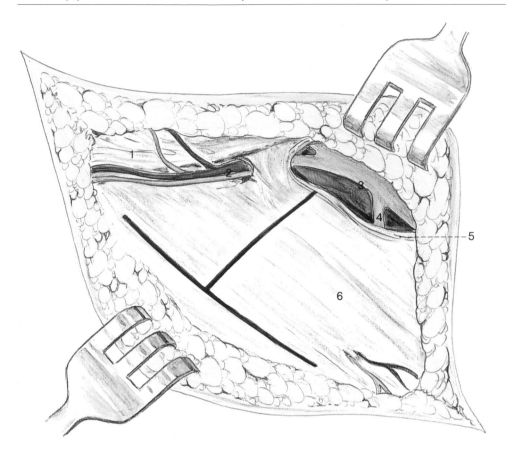

Fig. **273** For exposure of the nerve in the thigh, a T-shaped incision is made in the fascia lata

1 Inguinal ligament
2 Superficial circumflex iliac artery and vein
3 Femoral artery and vein
4 Great saphenous vein
5 Saphenous hiatus (margo falciformis)
6 Fascia lata

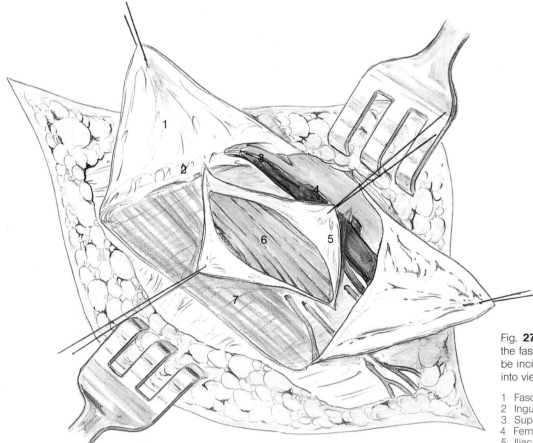

Fig. **274** After the T-shaped opening of the fascia lata, the iliac fascia, too, can now be incised so that the nerve is brought into view

1 Fascia lata with T-incision
2 Inguinal ligament
3 Superficial circumflex iliac artery and vein
4 Femoral artery and vein
5 Iliac fascia (incised)
6 Femoral nerve
7 Iliopsoas muscle with iliac fascia

Exposure in the Pelvic Region

(Figs. 275, 276)

Once the abdominal contents and investing adipose tissue have been adequately retracted medially, the femoral nerve appears in the angle between the iliac muscle and the lateral wall of the greater psoas muscle. It can be identified both by its course, in the direction of the inguinal ligament, and by its thickness.

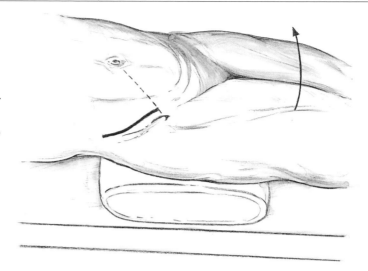

Fig. **275**   Incision for exposure of the femoral nerve in the pelvic region. *Dashed line:* line from the spinoumbilical line. *Arrow:* rotation of the thigh

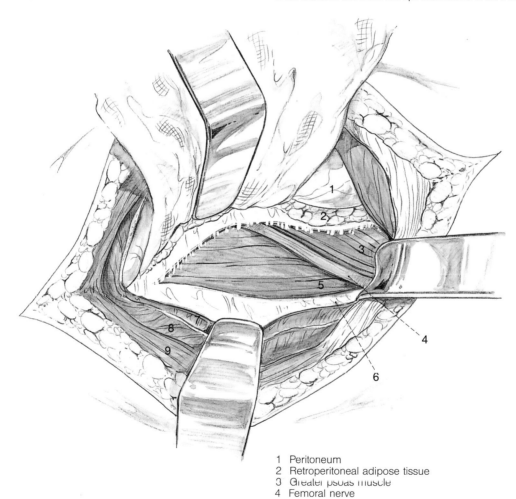

1 Peritoneum
2 Retroperitoneal adipose tissue
3 Greater psoas muscle
4 Femoral nerve
5 Iliac muscle
6 Transverse fascia
7 Transverse muscle of the abdomen
8 Internal oblique muscle of the abdomen
9 External oblique muscle of the abdomen

Fig. **276**   After layered opening of the abdominal wall, the transverse fascia can be incised, and the peritoneum with its contents can be retracted medially. The femoral nerve is visualized between the greater psoas muscle and the iliac muscle

Wound Closure

The fasciae are carefully closed. The same principle applies to the subcutaneous tissues and the skin.

Potential Errors and Dangers

— Injuries to the femoral vessels
— Overlooked injuries to the peritoneum and intestine

Approaches to the Obturator Nerve

Typical Indications for Surgery

- Abductor spasm (in some cases with simultaneous transection of the femoral nerve)
- Hip joint denervation in patients with chronic hip joint pain
- Rarely, injury cases

Principal Anatomical Structures

Medial border of greater psoas muscle, sacroiliac articulation, common iliac artery and vein, obturator foramen.

Positioning and Skin Incision
(Fig. 277)

The patient is placed in a supine position, and the ipsilateral pelvis is slightly underpadded. For intrapelvic extraperitoneal exposure, the skin incision is made at McBurney's point, just as in appendectomy. For exposure beneath the inguinal ligament, the incision is placed medial to the palpable femoral vessels and lateral to the adductors.

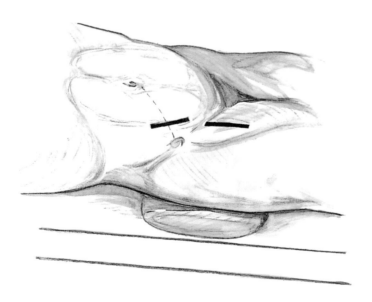

Fig. **277** Exposure of the obturator nerve in the pelvic region: positioning and incision. Also shown is the skin incision for exposure below the inguinal ligament (spinoumbilical line).

Dissection of Muscle Layers and Soft Tissues
(Fig. 278)

After the skin incision, the internal oblique muscle of the abdomen can be distracted in the direction of its fibers. The same procedure is followed with the transverse muscle of the abdomen. The subjacent transverse fascia is divided in the direction of the muscle fibers. After this, the peritoneum can be bluntly retracted medially. The external iliac artery and vein are now brought into view, and can be dissected free and subsequently retracted medially.

Exposure of the Nerve
(Fig. 279)

In the resulting gap between the wall of the lesser pelvis and the iliac vessels, the obturator nerve is visualized medial to the greater psoas muscle. From here, the femoral nerve, too, can be accessed lateral to the greater psoas muscle.

For operations below the inguinal ligament, the adductors have to be retracted medially and downward, so that the neurovascular bundle can be visualized. After this, the articular branches of the nerve can be identified by their course.

Wound Closure

Incised fasciae and muscles are carefully closed. Suture of subcutaneous tissues and skin completes the operation.

Potential Errors and Dangers

- Overlooked injuries to the iliac and femoral vessels
- Overlooked injury to the femoral nerve
- Overlooked injury to the peritoneum and intestine
- Abdominal hernias due to inadequate closure of the abdominal wall

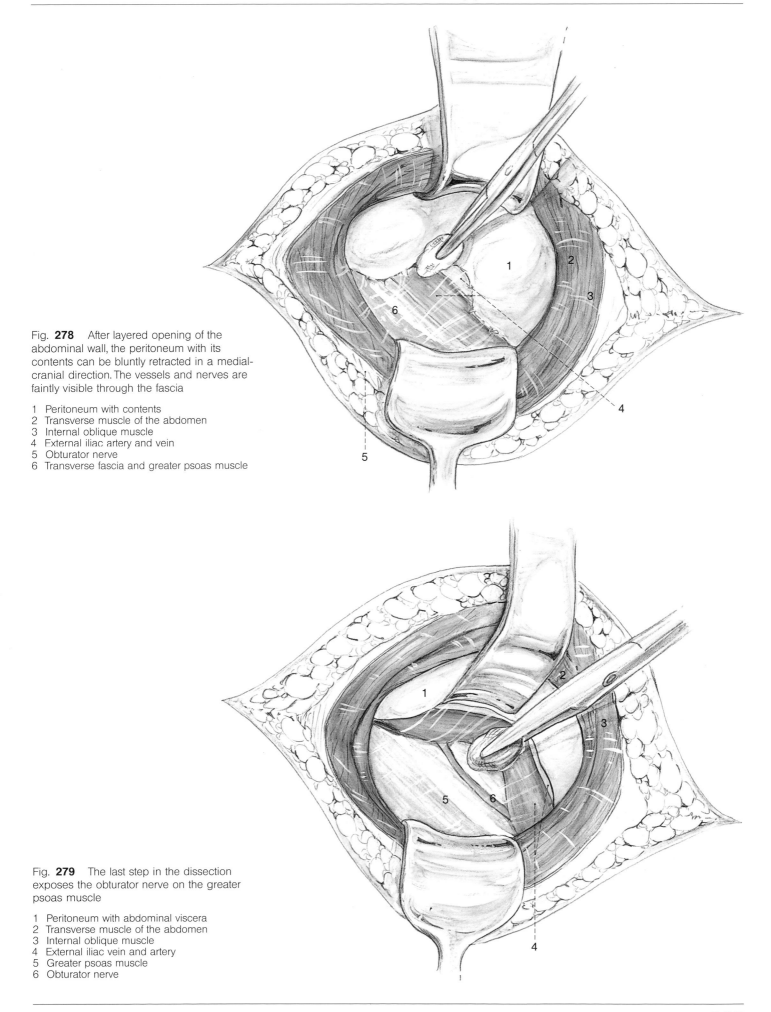

Fig. **278**   After layered opening of the abdominal wall, the peritoneum with its contents can be bluntly retracted in a medial-cranial direction. The vessels and nerves are faintly visible through the fascia

1   Peritoneum with contents
2   Transverse muscle of the abdomen
3   Internal oblique muscle
4   External iliac artery and vein
5   Obturator nerve
6   Transverse fascia and greater psoas muscle

Fig. **279**   The last step in the dissection exposes the obturator nerve on the greater psoas muscle

1   Peritoneum with abdominal viscera
2   Transverse muscle of the abdomen
3   Internal oblique muscle
4   External iliac vein and artery
5   Greater psoas muscle
6   Obturator nerve

Approaches to the Sciatic Nerve

Typical Indications for Surgery

— Direct injuries (stabbing, metal, gunshot)
— Indirect injuries (hematomas)
— Fractures (sacrum, ilium, femur)
— Dislocations (hip joint)
— Iatrogenic lesions (femoral neck operation, osteotomy, hip joint endoprosthesis)

Principal Anatomical Structures

Greater ischiadic foramen, piriform muscle, ischial bone, gluteus maximus, superior and inferior gemellus muscle, quadrate muscle of thigh, greater trochanter, femur, biceps muscle of thigh, adductor magnus muscle, semitendinous and semimembranous muscles.

Positioning and Skin Incisions
(Fig. 280)

The patient is placed in a prone position, and a soft pad is placed under the pelvis; the leg is externally rotated at the

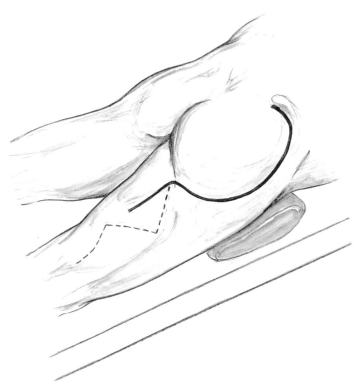

hip joint in order to relax the gluteal muscle. The posterior incision runs in an arc from the line connecting the coccyx with the iliac crest around the gluteal muscle, and into the gluteal fold. The distal skin incision for exposure of the nerve in the thigh follows the posterior midline of the thigh, beginning at the gluteal fold and extending distally for varying lengths.

Dissection of Soft Tissues in the Pelvis and Thigh
(Fig. 281)

After incision of the superficial fascia, the gluteus maximus muscle is partly exposed. Depending on the desired scope of exposure of the sciatic nerve, the procedure continues between the muscle fibers of the gluteus maximus or after its separation from the insertion. When passing between the muscle fibers, the nerve can be reached below the transversely coursing piriform muscle and on top of the superior and inferior gemellus muscles and the quadrate muscle of the thigh. The posterior cutaneous nerve of the thigh, which has to be spared, is situated somewhat more superficially and medially. If a greater exposed length of the nerve is required, the gluteus maximus muscle is detached at its fascia lata insertion, with enough tissue remaining on both sides for the final suture. Redissection of the muscle medially calls for special care in protecting numerous veins and arteries, particularly the median circumflex femoral artery and vein with the acetabular branch.

Exposure of the Nerve in the Pelvis
(Fig. 282)

The nerve is exposed to various lengths, depending on the approach used. Since localization of the damage to the sciatic nerve is not possible with sufficient precision because of the fiber distribution, the larger operation is found to be necessary more often than is initially assumed. The local anatomical situation is shown in the illustration. The smaller approach usually permits direct exposure only of the piriform muscle, the sciatic nerve, and the posterior cutaneous nerve of the thigh.

Fig. **280** Exposure of the sciatic nerve in the pelvic and femoral regions: positioning and incisions. *Dashed lines:* exposure in the gluteal region and thigh

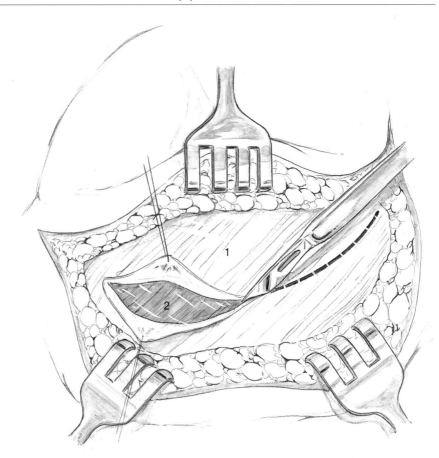

Fig. **281** The extensive skin incision is followed by incision of the fascia of the gluteus maximus muscle. *Red dashed line:* complete fascial incision

1 Fascia of gluteus maximus muscle
2 Gluteus maximus muscle

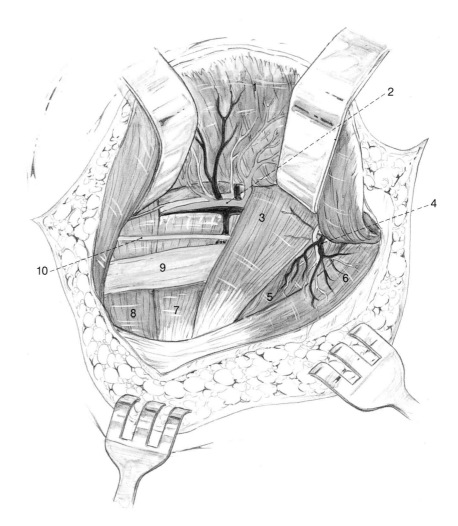

Fig. **282** Exposure of the nerve after division of the gluteus maximus muscle at its fascial insertion

1 Gluteus maximus
2 Inferior gluteal artery, vein, and nerve
3 Piriform muscle
4 Superior gluteal artery and vein
5 Gluteus minimus
6 Gluteus medius
7 Internal obturator muscle and gemellus muscles
8 Quadrate muscle of the thigh
9 Sciatic nerve
10 Posterior cutaneous nerve of the thigh

Exposure of the Nerve in the Thigh
(Figs. **283, 284**)

The superficial fascia, too, is divided longitudinally, again with care being taken to spare the posterior cutaneous nerve of the thigh. In the upper operative field, the inferior border of the gluteus maximus muscle has to be developed; after this, the biceps muscle of the thigh is the next principal muscle. In the upper regions of the thigh, the long head of the biceps muscle is retracted toward the middle, so that access can be gained to the sciatic nerve. In the middle segment of the thigh, this muscle is displaced laterally, so that the semitendinous and semimembranous muscles are found on the medial side of the exposed portions of the sciatic nerve.

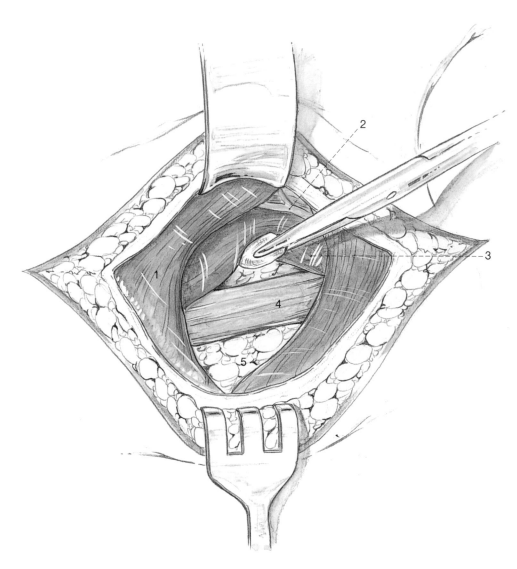

Fig. **283**   Exposure of the sciatic nerve directly beneath the vascular fold. The incision follows the longitudinal axis of the leg. The sciatic nerve appears deep to the medially retracted biceps muscle of the thigh

1 Gluteus maximus
2 Posterior cutaneous nerve of the thigh
3 Biceps muscle of the thigh (long head)
4 Sciatic nerve
5 Subgluteal adipose tissue

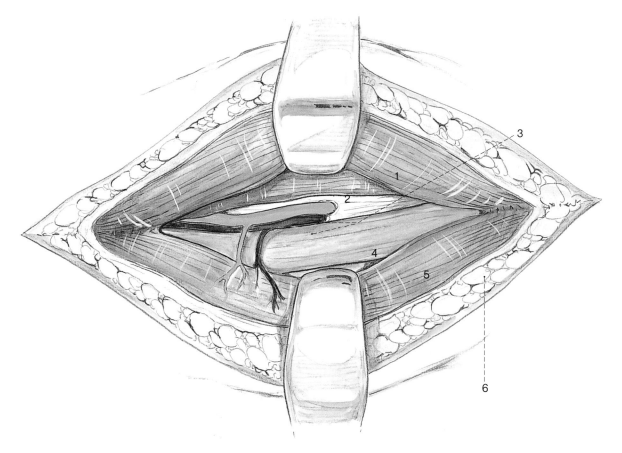

Fig. **284** Exposure of the sciatic nerve on the dorsal side of the thigh. The sciatic nerve can be exposed between the semitendinous muscle (medial) and the laterally situated biceps muscle of the thigh

1 Semitendinous muscle
2 Semimembranous muscle
3 Second perforating artery and vein
4 Sciatic nerve
5 Biceps muscle of thigh (long head)
6 Fascia lata

Wound Closure

Muscles that were divided in the course of the operation are approximated; muscles separated at their insertions, particularly the gluteus maximus, are carefully sutured. Fasciae should also be closed again. When suturing subcutaneous tissues and the skin, special care is taken to prevent contractile scar formation in junctional areas.

Potential Errors and Dangers

— Overlooked injury to adjacent nerves and vessels
— Overextension of nerves due to positioning or use of spatulas, or both
— Inadequate anchoring of the gluteus maximus due to an insufficiently sized zone of insertion

Approaches to the Tibial Nerve

Typical Indications for Surgery

Injuries occur here far less frequently than with the fibular nerve.

— Sharp injuries (glass, metal, gunshot)
— Blunt injuries
— Dislocations (tibia)
— Fractures (supracondylar femoral fracture, tibia)

Principal Anatomical Structures

Biceps muscle of the thigh, semitendinous and semimembranous muscles, heads of the gastrocnemius muscle, soleus muscle, popliteal muscle, medial border of the Achilles tendon, inner malleolus.

Positioning and Skin Incisions

With the patient in a prone position and the leg internally rotated at the hip by 45 degrees, the skin incision is made above the popliteal fossa between the biceps muscle of the thigh and the semitendinous and semimembranous muscles (Fig. 285). For the approach in the popliteal fossa, the incision – with the same positioning – is continued across the popliteal fossa and completed distally at right angles on the lateral border of the gastrocnemius muscle. In the lower leg region, exposure of the nerve is performed with the patient in a lateral position and the leg internally rotated. The skin incision (Fig. 286) descends from the lateral condyle and 3 cm behind the palpable tibial border in the direction of the inner malleolus. To expose the tibial nerve in the malleolar region (Fig. 287), the incision begins 8 cm above the inner malleolus and passes around it at right angles at a distance of 2 cm; it continues parallel to the first metatarsophalangeal joint. The patient is in a supine position, with the leg and foot abducted and externally rotated.

Dissection of the Tibial Nerve Above and Inside the Popliteal Fossa

(Fig. 288)

When dividing the fascia lata longitudinally, attention has to be paid first to the posterior cutaneous nerve of the thigh. Proceeding further, variously crosslinked veins are encountered in the subfascial adipose tissue. Within the adipose tissue of the popliteal fossa, the small saphenous vein, and below it the tibial nerve and the popliteal vein and artery, are reached. The muscular boundaries of the approach site are formed laterally by the biceps muscle of the thigh, the gastrocnemius muscle (lateral head), and the tendon of the plantar muscle, and medially by the semimembranous muscle, the gastrocnemius muscle (medial head), and the popliteal muscle.

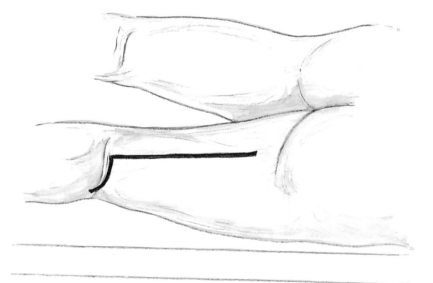

Fig. **285**   L-shaped exposure of the tibial nerve in the thigh

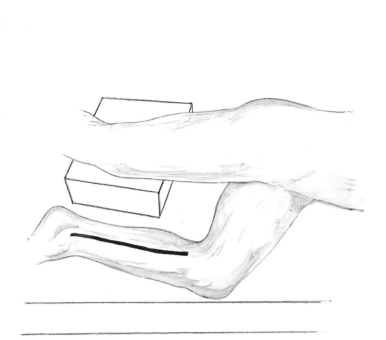

Fig. **286**   Incision for exposure of the tibial nerve in the lower leg

Fig. **287**   Incision for exposure of the tibial nerve at the ankle. *Dashed line:* extension

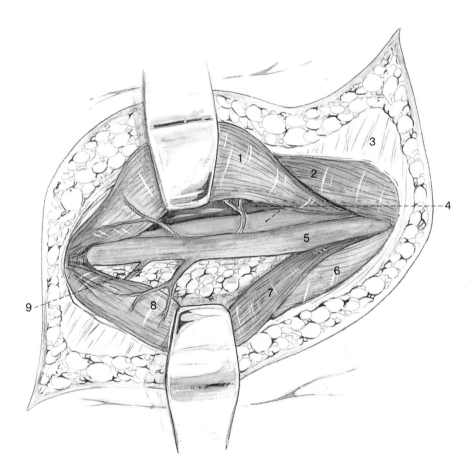

Fig. **288**   In the popliteal fossa, the nerve can be exposed below two investing muscle layers. The popliteal or tibial artery, which is readily palpable, can serve as landmark

1 Gastrocnemius muscle (medial head)
2 Semimembranous muscle
3 Fascia lata
4 Tibial artery and vein
5 Tibial nerve
6 Biceps muscle of the thigh
7 Gastrocnemius muscle (lateral head)
8 Soleus muscle
9 Sural nerve

Exposure of the Nerve in the Lower Leg
(Fig. **289**)

The superficial fascia is again divided longitudinally, accompanying veins being kept in sight. The muscle sulcus is bounded ventrally by the long flexor muscle of the toes and the posterior tibial muscle, and dorsally by the soleus muscle and the gastrocnemius muscle. Division of the deep crural fascia follows, and may be supplemented if necessary by incision or transection of the soleus muscle insertion. The neurovascular tract is now exposed (Fig. **290**).

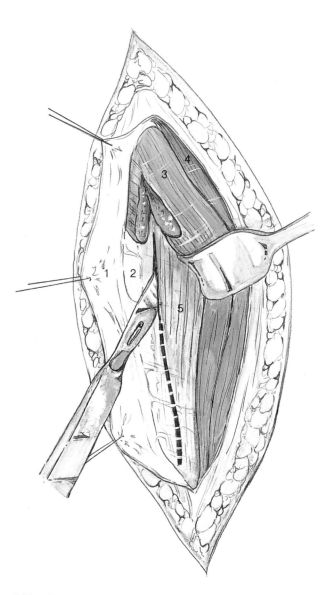

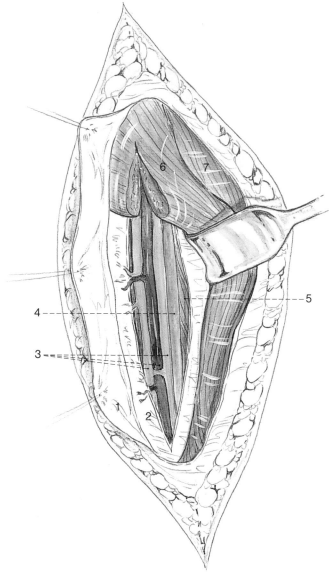

Fig. **289** For exposure of the tibial nerve in the leg, the soleus muscle has to be notched and the deep crural fascia longitudinally incised (dashed line)

1 Superficial crural fascia
2 Tibia
3 Soleus muscle (notched)
4 Gastrocnemius muscle
5 Deep crural fascia

Fig. **290** After this, the neurovascular bundle is exposed to the desired extent

1 Superficial crural fascia
2 Deep crural fascia
3 Posterior tibial veins and artery
4 Tibial nerve
5 Long flexor muscle of the great toe
6 Soleus muscle (notched)
7 Gastrocnemius muscle

Exposure of the Nerve at the Ankle
(Fig. 291)

Just below the divided superficial fascia, one finds the deep layer of the fascia, which is likewise divided in the direction of the skin incision. The neurovascular tract lies directly underneath. If the dissection is extended distally, the superficial layer of the flexor muscle retinaculum (ligamentum laciniatum) has to be divided.

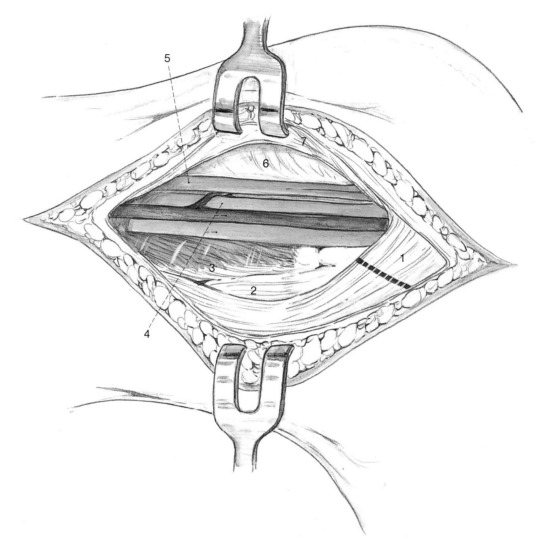

Fig. **291**   On the inner malleolus, division of the variously well-developed flexor retinaculum determines the extent to which the nerve can be exposed

1 Retinaculum of the flexor muscles (incision line)
2 Posterior tibial muscle
3 Long flexor muscle of the toes
4 Posterior tibial veins and artery
5 Tibial nerve
6 Crural fascia
7 Superficial fascia

Wound Closure

Notched and divided muscles and fasciae are reunited, close attention being paid to adjacent nerves and vessels. Oozing hemorrhages from the copiously crosslinked veins should be checked once again and arrested. The suture of subcutaneous tissues and skin requires special care, particularly on the lower leg and the ankle, and not infrequently calls for consideration of cosmetic aspects.

Potential Errors and Dangers

– Overlooked injury to adjacent nerves and vessels
– Inadequate suture of muscles and fasciae
– Inadequate protection of venous networks
– Excessive interruption of the crural venous system (edema)
– Insufficient skin closure, resulting in contractile scars

Approaches to the Peroneal Nerve (Fibular Nerve)

Typical Indications for Surgery

- Sharp injuries (glass, knife, iatrogenic)
- Blunt injuries
- Burns
- Fractures (femur, fibula)
- Dislocations (tibia, fibula)
- Plaster casts
- Sleep paralyses

Principal Anatomical Structures

Medial border of the tendon of the biceps muscle of the thigh, proximal and lateral borders of the popliteal fossa, popliteal fascia, head of the fibula, lateral surface of the fibula (superficial fibular nerve), medial surface of the fibula, and lateral border of the anterior tibial muscle (deep fibular nerve).

Positioning and Incisions

The patient is placed on the unaffected side, and the leg is internally rotated at the hip (Fig. 292); for exposure in the lower leg region, the supine position is used. In the area of the popliteal fossa, the incision begins at the medial border of the semitendinous muscle; it crosses the popliteal fossa in a lateral direction, and courses downward at the lateral border of the gastrocnemius muscle. Viewed in toto, the skin incision is Z-shaped. Depending on the scope of the exposure, longer or shorter longitudinal arms are employed. At the head of the fibula, the incision may curve concavely around the bony point, and may be continued downward if necessary. At the lower end of the lower leg, the incision is made parallel and lateral to the palpable ridge of the tibia (Fig. 293).

Exposure of the Nerve in the Knee Region
(Fig. 294)

The superficial fascia also receives a Z-shaped incision, the directly subjacent posterior cutaneous nerve of the thigh being spared. Cranial to the fibular head, the common fibular nerve can be exposed by mobilizing the medial border of the biceps muscle of the thigh; at the level of the palpable and visible fibular head, the nerve trunk that is immediately adjoining dorsally and caudally can be dissected free directly.

The surrounding fatty tissue detracts from the operative view.

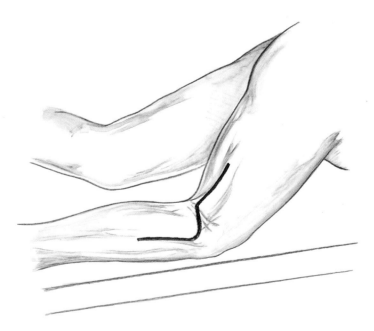

Fig. **292** Z-shaped exposure of peroneal nerve in the leg: positioning and incisions

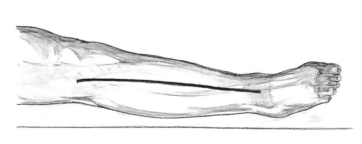

Fig. **293** Incision for exposure of the peroneal nerve in the lower leg

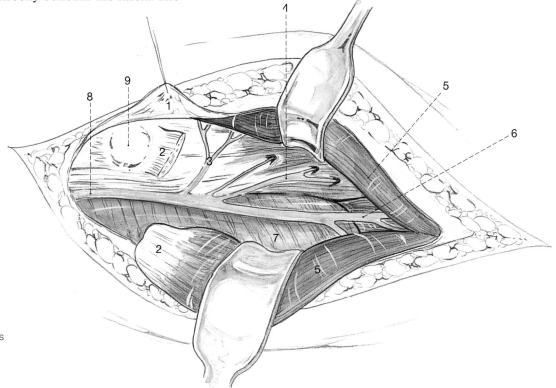

Fig. **294** The palpable fixation point for exposure of the nerve in the knee region is the head of the fibula, behind which the nerve is visualized (proximal lower leg region)

1 Superficial crural fascia
2 Soleus muscle
3 Posterior cutaneous nerve of the thigh
4 Common fibular nerve
5 Biceps muscle of the thigh
6 Head of the fibula
7 Deep fibular nerve
8 Superficial fibular nerve
9 Long peroneal muscle

Exposure of the Nerve in the Upper Part of the Lower Leg
(Fig. 295)

Continuing the skin incision, the superficial crural fascia is incised along the medial border of the biceps. Here particular caution is required, because the fibular nerve near the head of the fibula courses directly beneath the fascia. The severely flattened shape of the nerve at this location also makes identification somewhat more difficult. The adjacent muscle is the soleus. Following exposure in the region of the fibular head, it is necessary to decide whether all the branches of the fibular nerve need to be exposed. If so, the fibers of the fibular nerve that arise at the fibular head have to be divided.

Fig. **295** The further course of the nerve becomes visible after separation of the long peroneal muscle at the head of the fibula

1 Superficial crural fascia
2 Long peroneal muscle (detached)
3 Muscular branches of the long extensor muscle of the toes
4 Deep fibular nerve
5 Long extensor muscle of the toes
6 Superficial fibular nerve
7 Soleus muscle
8 Common fibular nerve
9 Head of fibula

Exposure of the Nerve in the Middle and Lower Portions of the Lower Leg
(Fig. 296)

In keeping with the situation of the nerve, an anterior approach is used in this nerve segment. The fascial incision corresponds to the longitudinal incision of the skin. The most medially located lower leg muscle, the anterior tibial muscle, is identified. After this, dissection in depth can be performed in the groove between the anterior tibial muscle and the laterally adjoining long extensor muscle of the great toe and the long extensor muscle of the toes.

The deep fibular nerve appears laterally from the anterior tibial blood vessels. Its principal visible branches run into the laterally situated extensors, but it innervates all the extensors.

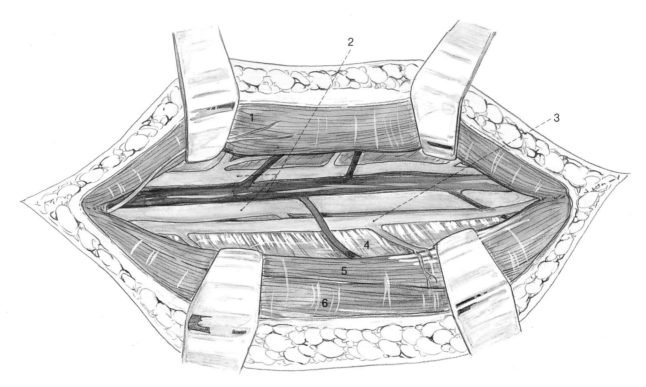

Fig. **296**   For exposure of the nerve in the middle and lower parts of the lower leg, the anterior tibial muscle and the long extensor muscles of the great toe and the toes are retracted

1 Anterior tibial muscle
2 Anterior tibial veins and artery
3 Deep fibular nerve
4 Interosseous membrane and posterior tibial muscle
5 Long extensor muscle of the great toe
6 Long extensor muscle of the toes

Wound Closure

The fasciae and notched or divided muscles are reunited. The closure of subcutaneous tissues and the skin of the lower leg and foot has to be done with special attention to cosmetic effects.

Potential Errors and Dangers

— Overlooked injury to adjacent nerves and vessels
— Overlooked persistent oozing hemorrhage from the venous plexus
— Excessive interruption of venous drainage conduits
— Inadequate skin closure

Approach to the Pudendal Nerve

Typical Indications for Surgery

— Rarely indicated on the whole
— Pudendal neuralgia
— Refractory pruritus ani and vulvae
— Refractory spastic states of the urethra

Principal Anatomical Structures

Piriform muscle, infrapiriform foramen, spine of the ischium, sacrotuberal ligament, sacrospinal ligament, internal obturator muscle, inferior gluteal vessels.

Positioning and Incision

(Fig. 297)

The patient lies prone, with the leg sharply rotated externally at the hip to relax the gluteus maximus muscle. The skin incision is made 4 cm below the middle and parallel to the so-called iliotrochanteric line (the connection between the tip of the greater trochanter and the posterior superior iliac spine; Fig. 297); it corresponds to the course of the piriform muscle.

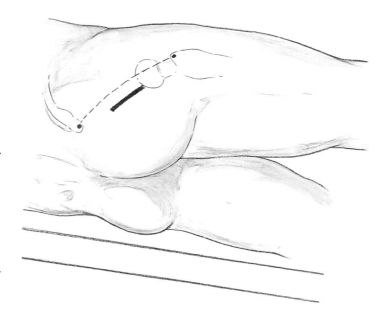

Fig. **297** Exposure of the pudendal nerve in the pelvic region: positioning and incision. The palpable points, the posterior superior iliac spine and the greater trochanter, as well as the dotted connecting line, are marked black

Dissection of Soft Tissues

(Fig. 298)

The fascia is divided in the direction of the skin incision. The subjacent fibers of the gluteus maximus muscle can be bluntly distracted (with index finger and small swabs). The fibers should run parallel to the skin incision; otherwise, the approach is placed too far cranially, and the middle gluteal muscle is encountered. After passage of the muscle, a layer of fatty tissue below the gluteus maximus is entered; in this layer, the ischiadic spine is again bluntly palpated at the inferior border of the piriform muscle. This area can then be explored with spatulas, so that the gliding surface between the gluteus maximus, on the one hand, and the gluteus medius muscle and the short hip muscles, on the other hand, can be incised.

Exposure of the Nerve

(Fig. 299)

The pudendal nerve, as well as the largest vessels in its immediate vicinity, are exposed under the fascia, which has been divided in line with the course of the nerve. The dissection therefore has to be carried out with extreme caution. The thick and readily palpable sciatic nerve lies lateral to the exposed structures.

Wound Closure

Following careful hemostasis, the subcutaneous tissue and the skin are sutured in layers. Whether to insert a drain depends on the extent of intraoperative bleeding.

Potential Errors and Dangers

— Injury to adjacent nerves and vessels due to instruments and excessive digital and spatula traction and pressure
— Overlooked oozing hemorrhages with consequent deep-seated hematoma (infection danger)
— Inappropriate wound closure

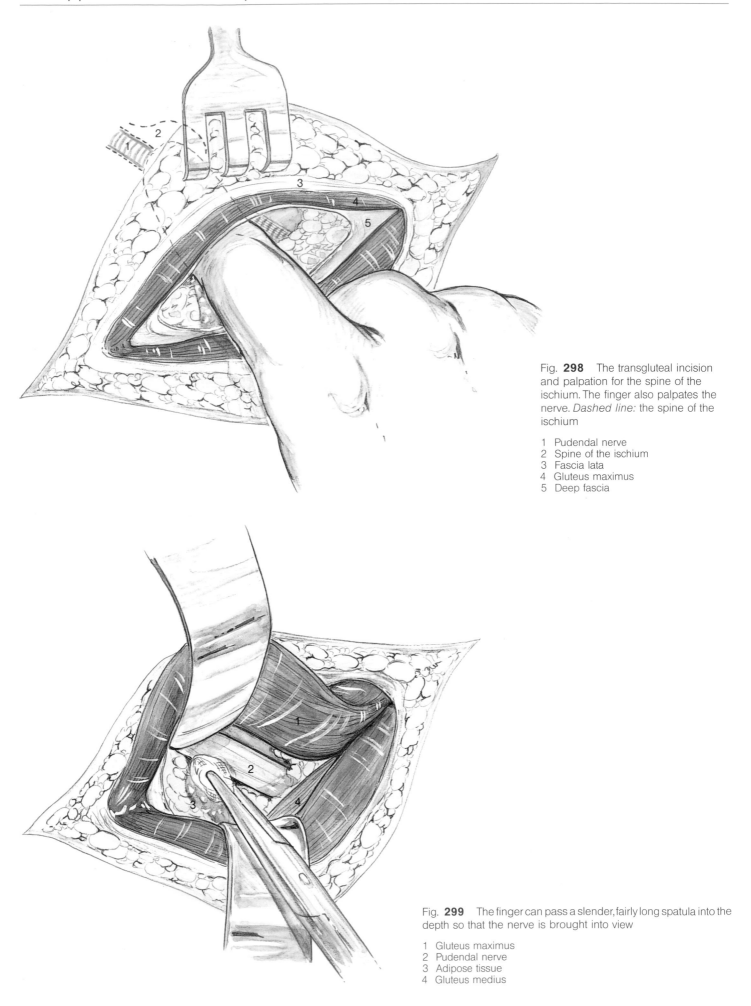

Fig. **298** The transgluteal incision and palpation for the spine of the ischium. The finger also palpates the nerve. *Dashed line:* the spine of the ischium

1 Pudendal nerve
2 Spine of the ischium
3 Fascia lata
4 Gluteus maximus
5 Deep fascia

Fig. **299** The finger can pass a slender, fairly long spatula into the depth so that the nerve is brought into view

1 Gluteus maximus
2 Pudendal nerve
3 Adipose tissue
4 Gluteus medius

Approaches to the Intercostal Nerves

Typical Indications for Surgery

— Intercostal neuralgia secondary to herpes zoster
— Neuralgias from local tumor infiltration
— Anastomoses to brachial nerves in brachial plexus pareses
— Harvesting of interposition material for nerve reconstruction

Principal Anatomical Structures

Inferior angle of the scapula, median axillary line, border of the greater rhomboid muscle, inferior costal margin.

Positioning and Skin Incisions

(Fig. **300**)

An overdrawn lateral position with anterior-superior abduction of the patient's arm is preferred. The degree of the lateral rotation depends on the location of the incision. The skin incision may be made parallel to the rib (1), parallel to the spine (2), or in the median axillary line (3). In some cases, a flap incision with its base on a rib is preferred. At the level of the first to fifth ribs, paravertebral approaches are precluded by the overlying scapula. For the harvesting of nerve interposition grafts, the area between the costal angle and the median axillary line is exposed.

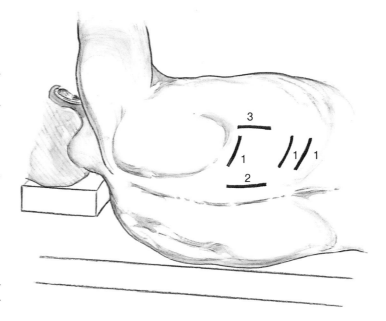

Fig. **300**   Exposure of the intercostal nerves: positioning and incisions

Dissection of Upper Muscle Layers
(Fig. **301**)

Depending on the level of the approach and its lateral location, muscle layers of varying thickness are included in the approach site. Mainly involved are the greater rhomboid muscle, the longissimus muscles of the neck and thorax, and the posterior inferior serratus muscle. The external intercostal muscle is then exposed.

Exposure of Nerve and Vessels
(Fig. **302**)

Depending on the desired extent of nerve exposure, blunt distraction of the external intercostal muscle may be sufficient, or a longer incision alongside the affected rib may be required. The nerve and vessel order is vein-artery-nerve, as seen in a caudal direction from a cranial viewpoint. The situation of the neurovascular bundle varies; near the vertebral column, it lies in the costal sulcus and is thus protected and covered by the rib; more laterally, the bundle lies in the middle of the intercostal space. Protection of the inner intercostal muscles and the adjoining pleura is vital.

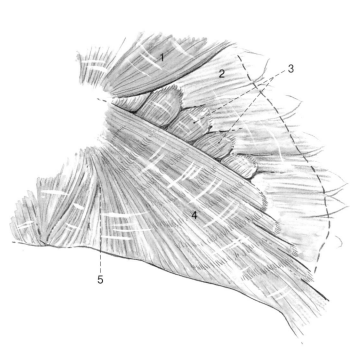

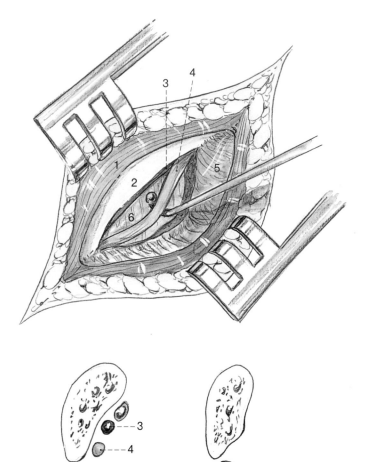

Fig. **301** Anatomical overview of the lateral superficial thoracic musculature

1 Greater pectoral muscle
2 External oblique muscle of abdomen
3 Anterior serratus muscle
4 Latissimus dorsi muscle
5 Inferior angle of the scapula

Fig. **302** An incision parallel to the inferior border of a rib, followed by division of the intercostal musculature. The two insets indicate the migration of the intercostal artery during its course from dorsal to ventral

1 Anterior serratus muscle
2 Rib
3 Intercostal artery
4 Intercostal nerve
5 External intercostal muscle
6 Internal intercostal muscle

Wound Closure

When any pleural injury has been ruled out by careful inspection, divided muscles and subcutaneous tissue and skin are closed in layers. A need for drainage is not uncommon.

Potential Errors and Dangers

— Injury to intercostal vessels
— Injury to the pleura
— Overlooked development of broadly expanded local hematomas

Approach to the Sural Nerve

Typical Indications for Surgery

— Collection of biopsy specimens in neuromuscular diseases
— Harvesting of interposition material for nerve replacement

Principal Anatomical Structures

Heads of the gastrocnemius muscle, accompanying small saphenous vein; occasionally, concomitant cutaneous artery; lateral malleolus.

Positioning and Incision

(Fig. **303**)

For the removal of biopsy material, the patient is placed in a prone position; for the harvesting of interposition grafts, the position is determined by the principal operative site. The leg is then internally rotated as far as possible.

Nevertheless, removal of the nerve tissue may still prove rather difficult. At times, it may even become necessary to reposition the patient during the operation. Time is saved by using separate surgical teams for the nerve operation, on the one hand, and for the harvesting of graft material, on the other. The distal skin incision is carried out 3–4 cm above the lateral malleolus and 3–4 cm outward from the lateral border of the Achilles tendon. Other transverse skin incisions are made over the course of the taut sural nerve.

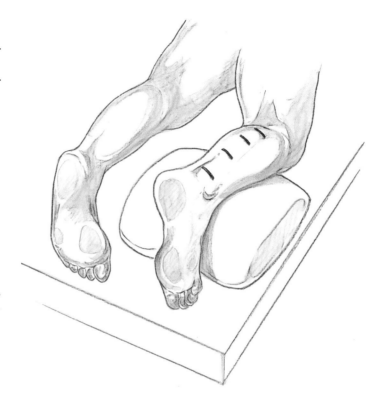

Fig. **303** Exposure of the sural nerve: positioning and incisions. The incisions run transverse to the course of the sural nerve

Identification of Nerve at Malleolus
(Fig. **304**)

After the skin incision described above, blunt dissection in the subcutaneous adipose tissue is used to localize the strong small saphenous veins and the sural nerve coursing parallel to it. The superficial crural fascia lies underneath. Traction on the snared nerve reveals its further course under the skin. In its uppermost visible segment, the nerve is once again exposed by a transverse incision 3–4 cm long; after distal separation, it is pulled out proximally, and the same procedure is carried out superiorly until interposition material of sufficient length becomes available. For biopsy, a one-time distal incision suffices.

Proximal Tracking of Nerves
(Fig. **305**)

The length of nerve that is visible through the skin should generally not be freed from the side branches of the nerve with a stripper. The use of slender grasping forceps and light traction is recommended instead. If this is not sufficient, additional transverse incisions are carried out. If the nerve disappears between the gastrocnemius heads, deeper dissection becomes necessary, but this is very rare.

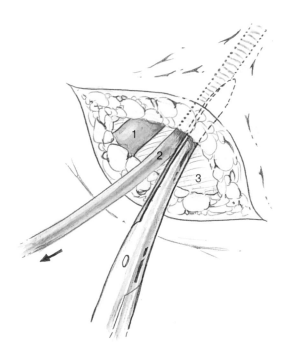

Fig. **304** After the small skin incision, it is usually the vein that is visualized to begin with; closely alongside, the nerve can be exposed and elevated on a tape, with its course ascertained

1 Small saphenous vein
2 Superficial crural fascia
3 Sural nerve (lateral dorsal cutaneous nerve)

Fig. **305** Tensioning the nerve aids further visualization of its proximal course, so that further transverse skin incisions can be kept short

1 Small saphenous vein
2 Sural nerve
3 Superficial crural fascia

Wound Closure

In conclusion, the subcutaneous tissue and the skin are closed after careful control of small hemorrhages.

Potential Errors and Dangers

– Failure to locate the sural nerve due to improper positioning
– Overlooked injury to adjacent peroneal areas
– Overlooked oozing hemorrhages covering wide areas

Index

Index